REACHING OUT TO CHILDREN
with FAS/FAE

*A Handbook for
Teachers, Counselors,
and Parents
Who Work with
Children Affected
by Fetal Alcohol
Syndrome & Fetal
Alcohol Effects*

DIANE DAVIS

THE CENTER FOR APPLIED
RESEARCH IN EDUCATION
West Nyack, New York 10995

10   9   8   7   6   5   4   3   2

Library of Congress Cataloging-in-Publication Data

Davis, Diane.
    Reaching out to children with FAS/FAE   :   a handbook for teachers, counselors, and parents who live and work with children affected by fetal alcohol syndrome & fetal alcohol effects / Diane Davis.
        p.   cm.
    Includes bibliographical references.
    ISBN 0–87628–857–3
    1. Children of prenatal alcohol abuse—Education—United States—Handbooks, manuals, etc.   2. Children of prenatal alcohol abuse—United States—Development—Handbooks, manuals, etc.   3. Fetal alcohol syndrome—United States—Handbooks, manuals, etc.
I. Center for Applied Research in Education.   II. Title.
LC4806.4.D38   1994
371.92—dc20
                                                                              94–11953
                                                                              CIP

ISBN 0-87628-857-3

THE CENTER FOR APPLIED
RESEARCH IN EDUCATION
Career & Personal Development Division
A division of Simon & Schuster

West Nyack, New York 10995

Printed in the United States of America

Eileen Ishizawa

This book is dedicated with love to

LINDA AND DANNY

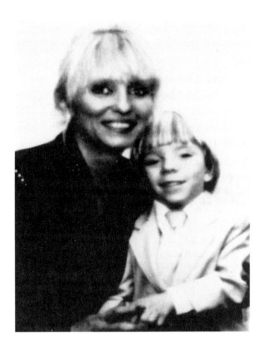

Danny, 5-1/2 years old with his mother.

About the Author

Diane Davis is a Certified Chemical Dependency Counselor, Consultant, and Educator who has worked with children and their families in a variety of therapeutic settings for over ten years. Her areas of expertise include domestic violence, chemical dependency, and fetal alcohol syndrome, and she is the author of *Something Is Wrong At My House* (Parenting Press, 1984) and *Working With Children From Violent Homes* (Network Publications, 1986). She has also served as adjunct faculty to numerous colleges in the Northwest, and is a popular trainer and workshop presenter at conferences. Ms. Davis received her master's degree in Psychology from Antioch University, Seattle, Washington.

Acknowledgments

I would like to take this opportunity to thank Dr. Ann Streissguth, Dr. Donna Burgess, and Sandra Randels, RN, MSN, for the many things I learned from them as I began my work in the field of fetal alcohol syndrome and its prevention.

I would also like to thank Michael Dorris for writing the book *The Broken Cord,* which spoke to so many thousands of people about what it is like to love and raise a child with FAS.

Over the past three years I have grown close to Jocie, Vicky, and Linda, three mothers who have children with either FAS or FAE and whose commitment to their children and to educating others about FAS/FAE has been astounding. I thank them for the love, encouragement and support they have always given me, especially throughout the various stages of my writing this book.

I also greatly appreciate the contributions of Dr. Michael Donlan, Dr. Lew Abrams, Marceil Ten Eyck, MC, CCDCII, Sydney Helbock, and Linda LaFever. I value their work and their words of wisdom and feel honored that they agreed to let me include their articles and their stories.

For me, writing a book is like taking a journey. Mid-way through the *Reaching Out* journey, Mary McConnon joined me to share with me her knowledge of computers, layout and graphics. Thank you, Mary, for your many hours of fine work and the hundreds of words you transcribed for me. I would have been lost without you!

I also want to thank my editor, Susan Kolwicz. She saw the promise in my original manuscript and guided me with her expertise, patience and sensitivity, as the manuscript grew into a book that I am very proud of.

Finally, I want to say "Thank you and I love you" to Karen Appelman, my friend since childhood, for being so instrumental in my life during the writing and publishing of this book. I will be forever grateful for your friendship, your support, and your ongoing belief in me.

Diane Davis

CHAPTER 4: TEACHING THE CHILD WITH FAS/FAE—37

SECTION II
TECHNIQUES FOR WORKING WITH CHILDREN, ADOLESCENTS, AND ADULTS WITH FAS/FAE

CHAPTER 5: TECHNIQUES FOR HELPING CHILDREN THROUGH ADULTS—67

CHAPTER 6: THE NEEDS OF OLDER CHILDREN WITH FAS/FAE—115

CHAPTER 7: FOR PARENTS AND COUNSELORS WITH ADOLESCENTS AND ADULTS WITH FAS/FAE —137

SECTION III
ARTICLES AND OTHER RESOURCES

Section I

The Child with FAS/FAE

*I*f you are the parent or teacher of a child with Fetal Alcohol Syndrome (FAS) or Fetal Alcohol Effects (FAE), no doubt you have faced many challenges. Although research on FAS/FAE has been going on for years and continues to progress, it is only recently that we have begun to come up with specific, concrete techniques to use with children with FAS/FAE and their families. These techniques help to reduce some of the frustrations that so many teachers and families with children with FAS/FAE experience. They can be expanded upon or modified to fit the needs of those who use them. There are no clear-cut answers as to "what works" for every child with FAS/FAE, but there are positives that we can build upon, and there is hope. This book has been written to educate those who are open to learning more about children with FAS/FAE and to offer support and hope to families who must deal with the reality of Fetal Alcohol Syndrome and Fetal Alcohol Effects on an ongoing basis in their lives.

CHAPTER 1

Diagnosis and Prognosis

What Is Fetal Alcohol Syndrome?

Fetal Alcohol Syndrome is the number one cause of mental retardation in our country today. Unlike Spina Bifida and Down Syndrome, the other two leading birth defects in the United States, FAS is totally preventable. The only way a child can be born with Fetal Alcohol Syndrome or Fetal Alcohol Effects is if the mother drinks alcohol during her pregnancy. Any alcohol taken in by the mother passes through the placenta and is also taken in by the fetus. If the mother gets drunk, so does her unborn child.

There is no known "safe" amount of alcohol for pregnant mothers to drink; therefore it is strongly advised that there be no drinking at all during pregnancy, including three months prior to conception. Different women metabolize (break down) alcohol at different rates in their bodies. Thus, some fetuses can be more affected than others by their mother's drinking.

If a mother's drinking increases over the years, the chance of her having children with Fetal Alcohol Effects

(FAE) and then Fetal Alcohol Syndrome (FAS) may also increase. For instance, her first child may be born with only slight effects and may even seem completely normal; her second child may have FAE; and her third child may have FAS. If the drinking stops after the third child, the mother's fourth child will not have FAE or FAS. Research about the impact of a father's drinking on the unborn child is still in the early stages.

Children with FAE may look perfectly normal and also have normal IQs, but their behaviors are very similar to those of children with FAS. Parents of children with FAE have also reported that many of their children have been slow in their physical development and tend to have learning disabilities.[1]

Presently, one in every 500 to 700 babies born in the United States is a Fetal Alcohol Syndrome baby. One in 300 to 350 has Fetal Alcohol Effects. In regions where there is a high rate of alcoholism and women who drink, the ratio can be as high as one in 100 babies being born with FAS.[2]

How to Distinguish FAS and FAE

A diagnosis needs to be made by a trained professional who understands FAS/FAE and knows exactly what to look for and what questions to ask. The diagnostician is generally a person with a medical degree who specializes in birth defects and has specific training in diagnosing FAS. When diagnosing a child as FAS, a trained expert looks for the following:

1. **Specific facial features.** These include:

❑ Small head size

❑ A flat midface and nasal bridge

---

[1] A.P. Streissguth and R.A. LaDue, "Fetal Alcohol: Teratogenic Causes of Developmental Disabilities," *Toxic Substances and Mental Retardation* (Washington, D.C.: American Association on Mental Deficiency, 1987), p. 68.

[2] Carole T. Giunta and Ann P. Streissguth, "Patients with Fetal Alcohol Syndrome and Their Caretakers," *The Journal of Contemporary Social Work,* 1988, pp. 453–459.

❏ Small eyes—the eyeslits may be short (normal eyeslits are equal in length to the length of the bridge of the nose)

❏ The absence of a ridge between the nose and the upper lip

❏ In some cases, the forehead may protrude and/or the chin may be pointed

2. **Growth deficiency** (smaller height and weight at birth)

3. **Damage to the central nervous system** (often causing mental retardation)

The diagnostician will take measurements of the child's head and face and make note of his or her height, weight, and other physical characteristics (such as apparent physical deformities). Because some ethnic groups tend to have flat faces and almond-shaped eyes, it is essential that a diagnosis be done by a professional who knows how to measure the face correctly. Also, as children get older, their facial features may change. Therefore, the earlier a child can be diagnosed, the better. (See Figure 1 and accompaying photos on pages 6–8.)

Figure 1.
FACES IN FETAL ALCOHOL SYNDROME

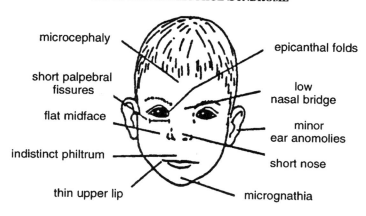

microcephaly

epicanthal folds

short palpebral fissures

low nasal bridge

flat midface

minor ear anomolies

indistinct philtrum

short nose

thin upper lip

micrognathia

Little & Streissguth, Unit 5, "Alcohol, Pregnancy, and Fetal Alcohol Syndrome," of *Alcohol Use and Its Medical Consequences*. (Timonium, MD: Milner, Fenwick, Inc., 1982).

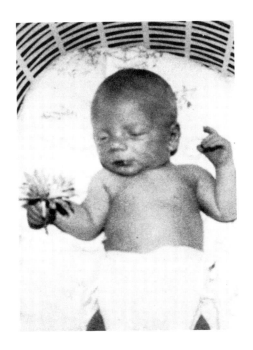

5 Days Old

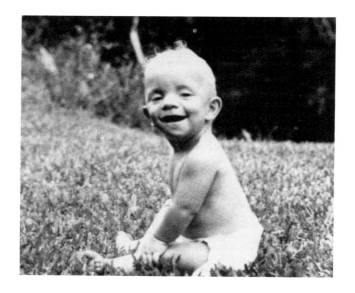

10 Months Old

Absence of philtrum, thin upper lip, protruding forehead, small eyes, flat nasal bridge, long chin.

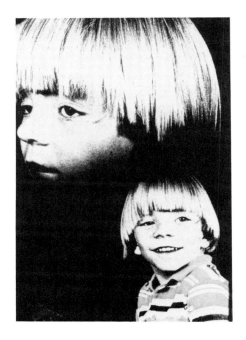

4-1/2 Years Old

Questions will be asked about the child's development over the years, and his behaviors. The diagnostician will also want to know how much alcohol and other drugs the mother consumed during her pregnancy. The exam itself does not take more than half an hour unless additional testing is advised. However, a specialist who diagnoses FAS or FAE is very thorough and considers a range of factors before making an absolute diagnosis.

A child with FAE has *two* of the *three* characteristics. Often the characteristic that is missing is the "Special Facial Features." Because many children with FAE look like all the other students, they are at high risk of "falling

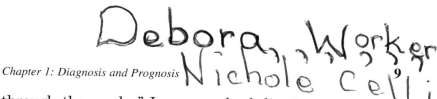

through the cracks." In some school districts, nurses are being trained to do initial screenings of students suspected to have FAS or FAE. If it seems fairly certain that the child has FAS or FAE, a recommendation needs to be made to the parents that the child be diagnosed by a trained physician.

Who Can Provide a Diagnosis?

Finding an expert to diagnose FAS may not always be easy. If you live in a large city, your pediatrician may be able to refer you to one. You may also check with a large hospital or university closest to where you live. They may have Child Evaluation Centers where your child can be fully assessed by a geneticist, dysmorphologist, or other specialists in birth defects. See the article by Dr. M. Donlan on page 149 for more information about the FAS/FAE diagnosis.

What Is the Advantage of a Diagnosis?

For most, the advantage of a diagnosis is that it is an answer—an explanation as to why a child has acted and reacted in certain ways. It can be a catalyst for parents to:

❏ Seek additional education and information

❏ Begin a process of personal recovery and healing for the mother and her family

❏ Have more information and a "label" to take to their child's school so that the child will (hopefully) get more help with her education

❏ Motivate families to get involved in educating the public about FAS/FAE and lobbying for more local, state and federal moneys for prevention and family assistance programs

What if Getting a Diagnosis Isn't Possible?

There are usually three main reasons why a family may not be able to get a diagnosis:

❑ No trained expert in their area

❑ The expert has a long waiting list

❑ Not enough history available on the birth mother (this is often the case when adoptive parents want a diagnosis)

When it isn't possible to get a diagnosis, parents will have to work closely with their child's school to get the school to provide whatever services are available for students with academic and/or behavior difficulties. Even if the child's IQ is too high for Special Education services, there are techniques and strategies that can be used both at school (in and outside the classroom) and at home that will benefit the child. (See the *Techniques* section for specific suggestions.) As more research is done and FAS/FAE is better understood by our society, getting a diagnosis should become easier and more services should be readily available to children with FAS/FAE and their families.

When Should FAS/FAE Be Suspected?

Along with the three main characteristics discussed earlier—specific facial features, growth deficiency, and damage to the central nervous system—the following traits indicate that a child needs to be evaluated for FAS/FAE.

Infants

❑ May smell like alcohol at birth and/or have tremors

❑ Irritable

❑ Poor sucking ability

❑ Can't tolerate much stimulation

❑ Slow in development

Toddlers and Preschoolers

❑ Can be lethargic or hyperactive

❑ Demand lots of one-on-one attention

❑ No sense of boundaries

❑ Have trouble learning right from wrong

❑ Often want lots of physical contact

❑ Lack of fear which can cause them to get into high-risk situations

❑ Poor memory

Grade School

❑ Continue to need lots of one-on-one attention

❑ Unable to stay on task

❑ Easily distracted/distracts others

❑ Poor coordination

❑ Poor judgment

❑ Can read and write, but tend to be slow

❑ Low social skills

❑ Can become easily upset (temper tantrums, crying, poor anger control)

Middle School

❑ Inability to keep up academically and socially

❑ Low self-esteem due to being rejected by others, so many failures, and the knowledge that they are different

❑ They need to "fit in" somewhere so they fall in with the wrong crowd—may lie, steal, cheat, fight, etc.

❑ They may have little or no concept of right or wrong

❑ Poor judgment

❑ Lack of fear

High School

❑ Getting into trouble and/or becoming a victim escalates

❑ Sex drive is usually normal, but impulse control is low or non-existent

❑ Little concept of how to handle money

❑ Basic living skills and hygienic needs may have to be taught over and over

❑ A primary caretaker may be needed to monitor the child with FAS/FAE, even when he becomes an adult

❑ Low ability to take care of own hygienic needs

Adults with FAS/FAE

Children never "outgrow" the damage of FAS/FAE as of this writing. Even though they grow to have adult bodies, emotionally those with FAS may remain very childlike (about seven or eight years of age). Early studies on adolescents and adults yielded results such as:

❑ The average IQ of a child or adult with FAS is 68.

❑ Academically, children may not progress beyond

second-third grade level in math

third-grade level in spelling

fourth-grade level in reading

As more children are diagnosed and their progress followed, however, these statistics are changing. Some children may perform very well at certain tasks and fail consistently at others. It is important to keep in mind that each child is different.

CHAPTER 2

Confronting the Cause: Alcoholism

"No one ever told me it would harm my baby if I drank during pregnancy," is something I have heard over and over again from biological mothers. Lack of education on the part of mothers and their doctors, as well as the denial, minimization, and rationalization that is characteristic of the disease of alcoholism, have all contributed to the drinking that produces children with FAS/FAE.

In 1976 the American Medical Society on Alcoholism published the following definition of alcoholism:

> Alcoholism is a chronic, progressive, and potentially fatal disease. It is characterized by: tolerance of and physical dependency to alcohol, pathologic organ changes, or both, all of which are the direct or indirect consequences of the alcohol ingested.[3]

---

[3] James E. Royce, Alcohol Problems and Alcoholism (New York: The Free Press, 1981), p. 15.

If the Birth Mother Is Still Drinking

If the birth mother is still drinking she is to some degree emotionally unavailable to her children. There may be physical, emotional, and/or sexual abuse going on, as well as general neglect. Children with FAS/FAE require constant nurturing and monitoring. They don't often get this from a mother who is an active alcoholic.

Instead of being harshly judged for their drinking, biological mothers need help to stop it if it is still occurring, and compassion and therapeutic support as they work through the guilt and shame they feel because of what has happened to their children. Family members and other adults involved with the family can participate in the recovery process of the biological mother by acknowledging and praising her willingness to get better.

Because of the drinking in the family, unhealthy roles and rules continue to be played out. It is essential that any abuse and neglect be reported to child protective authorities. Ideally, the mother will be ordered to get help for her alcoholism and all family members will receive counseling. In order for healing to take place—especially when an alcoholic mother is deep into denial—some kind of intervention must occur.

Understanding Family Dynamics

All family members are affected when alcoholism is present. Research shows that in order for these families to survive, they establish rules and roles that ultimately cause destructive patterns and behaviors. All members within the family follow rules that may either be spoken or unspoken. The rules in an alcoholic family include: "deny," "don't talk," "don't feel," "don't trust," "isolate." The roles in an alcoholic family include:

❏ The Abuser—the person who abuses alcohol

❏ The Co-Dependent or Enabler—the partner who puts up with the alcoholic behavior

❧ THE RULES IN AN ALCOHOLIC FAMILY ❧

DENY

that there is anything wrong

DON'T TALK

to each other or anyone outside the family about what is going on

DON'T FEEL

feelings are too threatening because they need to be dealt with

DON'T TRUST

especially anyone outside the family

ISOLATE

keep all the problems within the family

❧ THE ROLES IN AN ALCOHOLIC FAMILY ❧

THE ABUSER

THE CO-DEPENDENT OR ENABLER

THE HERO

THE SCAPEGOAT

THE FAMILY ANGEL

THE CLOWN/MASCOT

❑ The Hero—often the first-born child. This person may be the surrogate parent to younger siblings, is responsible, possibly an overachiever, the child who "makes the family look good"

❑ The Scapegoat—the troublemaker. Calls attention to the family's problems by "being such a problem." Rebellious, underachiever, etc.

❑ The Family Angel—seldom causes any trouble or "makes any waves." Compliant, passive, may be withdrawn or seem to be in "their own little world"

❑ The Clown/Mascot—distracts the family when problems arise by being clever, cute, funny, etc.

Family roles can change when there is a death, divorce, new addition to the family, someone leaves home, two families blend together, etc. Alcoholic families tend to need these roles to be filled and played out, whereas in healthy families, individuality is encouraged and feelings and situations are dealt with openly, as they occur. These rules and roles can be passed on from generation to generation.

What to Do with Feelings

Feelings in families where there is FAS or FAE can run very high. Parents may experience rage, guilt, shame, sadness, fear, confusion, frustration, hopelessness, and helplessness. Their other children may feel exactly the same emotions. It is important that family members learn to identify what emotions they are feeling and to find ways to appropriately express these emotions. Physically releasing energy and then talking feelings over with caring, supportive adults can prove to be very beneficial. Doing so requires breaking the *Deny, Don't Talk, Don't Feel,* and *Don't Trust* rules. It also helps to put an end to isolation and opens a family up to discovering new ways of handling things.

However, adults and older children often resist seeking outside help and insist that they can "manage their problems on their own." If you are a counselor, social worker or teacher working with such a family, you might ask them, "Have the ways you've been trying to manage them so far been working?" Their answer is usually "No."

Explain that raising a child with FAS/FAE is a constant challenge. It is also a full-time job. Reaching out to others for support and guidance can help relieve the feelings of helplessness, frustration, and feeling all alone. It can also provide an opportunity to learn new ways of parenting a child with FAS/FAE.

Recovery and Treatment Programs

When a family member is unhealthy, the whole family is impacted. Even if the alcoholic has stopped drinking, it is important that she follow a recovery program that nurtures and empowers her physically, emotionally and spiritually. A strong recovery program often includes:

Physical:

❑ Abstaining from the use of alcohol (and other drugs)

❑ Establishing healthy eating habits

❑ Getting enough rest

❑ Exercising regularly

Emotional:

❑ Attending Alcoholics Anonymous and/or other groups for chemically dependent people for understanding and emotional support

❑ Getting individual and/or group counseling with a professional trained to work with alcoholic clients

❑ Forming a healthy network of friends, family members and professionals who support the alcoholic's sobriety. (Often, AA and other twelve-step meetings are where friends are made)

❑ Obtaining a sponsor (a recovering alcoholic with several years of sobriety) to help guide the alcoholic in her recovery process

Spiritual:

❑ Seeking a deeper meaning in life whether it be through the belief in God or a higher power

❑ Striving toward empowering oneself

❑ Working the twelve steps that are taught in Alcoholics Anonymous and other meetings that support sobriety

Treatment Programs

Alcoholism is a disease that can cause much destruction. An alcoholic may need to enter a treatment program that provides both intensive education about this disease, as well as individual and group counseling. There are two kinds of treatment programs: inpatient (where the client lives at the treatment facility for a specific number of days) and outpatient (where the client attends educational and counseling sessions on a regular basis at an outpatient facility).

Treatment programs for alcoholics are usually listed in the phone book under alcoholism or chemical dependency. Often the larger treatment centers offer informational meetings that explain the treatment method they use, the duration of stay, what the client's daily routine will be, the cost of treatment, etc. The treatment center may also have Intervention Specialists on staff who coach family members and concerned others on how to confront the alcoholic in such a way that she will be motivated to follow through with treatment. (The Intervention Specialist is present and helps to facilitate the intervention when it occurs.)

The Rest of the Family

Just as an alcoholic needs to participate in a recovery process, so must other family members. Al-Anon is a program that is for adults who are and have been affected by an alcoholic's drinking. Ala-Teen is for teenagers with an alcoholic parent(s). KLUE (Kids Like Us are Everywhere) groups are for elementary-aged children who must deal with alcoholism in the home (KLUE groups are often offered in school settings) and Ala-Tot groups are also for young children from alcoholic homes. Codependency (CODA) groups can also be beneficial.

To find out what is available in your area, consult your phone book or call your local drug/alcohol hotline, crisis clinic or community services number. Family members deserve help and support. It is available and the groups listed above do not cost anything to attend. For more in-depth needs, individual or group therapy is advised.

Resources for Better Understanding Alcoholism and Its Effects on the Family

Three books that I highly recommend to those who want to better understand alcoholism and how it affects the family include:

James R. Milam, Ph.D., and Katherine Ketcham, *Under the Influence* (New York: Bantam Books, 1981).

John Bradshaw, *The Family* (Deerfield Beach, Florida: Health Communications, Inc., 1987).

Claudia Black, *It Will Never Happen to Me* (New York: Ballantine Books, 1981).

See the Readings section for additional books available on this subject.

CHAPTER 3

Parenting a Child with FAS/FAE

Infants with FAS/FAE may have a very hard time during their first few months. Many of them are unable to "screen out" all the stimulation around them. They can be irritable, and their poor coordination and sucking reflexes contribute to nursing difficulties. They can become easily frustrated because they can't get the nourishment they need (which is crucial because of their low birth weights). (See pages 22–24 on the stages of human development.)

It is recommended that these infants not be exposed to too much stimulation, especially when they are fed. Feeding them in a dark, quiet room and not rocking or talking to them will help them focus on sucking. You may also want to keep them wrapped in a blanket as this often helps to calm them.

It may be difficult to accept this method since there has been so much emphasis in recent years on talking to, touching, and smiling at the infant, as well as exposing him or her to bright colors, objects, and a variety of sounds and everyday activities. The child with FAS/FAE may be too sensitive to function in such a stimulating environment. He needs a calming atmosphere and a parent/caretaker who can be patient and let him nurse at his own pace. Gradually, stim-

STAGES OF HUMAN DEVELOPMENT

CONCEPTION - IMPLANTATION		EMBRYONIC STAGES IN WEEKS							FETAL STAGE	FULL TERM
1	2	3	4	5	6	7	8	9	Weeks 10–36	Weeks 38–42
		Brain Spine Heart	Heart Eyes Arms Legs	Eyes Heart Arms Legs	Eyes Ears Teeth	Palate	Palate Genitalia	Genitalia		

Central Nervous System
Heart
Arms
Legs
Eyes
Ears
Teeth
Palate
External Genitalia

Stages of development of major organs and the developmental periods when they are most likely to be damaged by teratogens. The solid bar is the most sensitive period of development.

DEVELOPMENTAL STAGES

Birth to 1 Month: Eats frequently, sucks, swallows, turns face toward or away from object, finger grasping.

2 Months: Adjusts to a regular routine, follows objects with eyes, responds to human face with a smile, raises head slightly.

3 Months: Smiles and coos, attracted by bright colors, moves head when following objects with eyes, can turn from side to side, can lift head and chest when on stomach, movements with arms and thrashing movements with legs.

4 Months: Recognizes mother, more eye-body coordination, likes to repeat acts, plays with hands and feet, rolls from stomach to back, sits up for brief periods of time when propped.

5 Months: Smiles at familiar faces, holds up arms to be picked up, continues to repeat acts which interest him, focuses on brightly moving objects, makes various sounds, plays with fingers and studies them intently, picks things up, can stay sitting up for longer periods of time when propped, rolls from back to stomach, can go longer (four to five hours) between meals.

6-7 Months: Is aware of familiar people and becomes afraid of strangers, babbles to self, reaches for objects, can sit erect for long periods of time, grasps, holds onto, and lets go of objects, puts everything in mouth.

8-9 Months: Begins to enjoy games like "pat-a-cake" and "peeka-boo," starts to link words with ideas and also imitates sounds, can pull self into a sitting position, begins to crawl on stomach, first teeth begin to come in.

10-11 Months: Likes lots of freedom—gets cranky if confined for more than brief periods, begins to say a few simple words, likes to push or bang objects together, creeps on all fours, may be able to pull self up to standing position, several teeth have now come through.

12 Months: Gets angry when objects are removed from view, understands more words, can put pegs into holes, is learning to stand alone and may take a few steps and sit himself down on the floor.

1-2 years: Walks alone, climbs stairs, drinks from cup, uses spoon, turns pages of a book, has vocabulary of 3–200 words and is able to say short sentences, may begin to use the word "No!" as he is beginning to learn to assert his independence, shows strong feelings of anger and frustration, still needs help getting dressed and undressed.

3 years: Walks and runs easily, asks "Why?" frequently, begins to understand number concepts, vocabulary is now 800–900 words, starts to recognize and identify colors, begins to understand cause and effect, can ride a tricycle, is beginning to be able to put clothes on and take them off with limited help.

4 years: Is able to cooperate when playing with two or three others, understands simple reasons for things, has a vocabulary of approximately 1,500 words, knows her age, knows how to compare, can be argumentative, dresses self.

5 years: Understands rules and can explain them to others, can now play in larger groups, knows name and address, drawings become more recognizable, frequently asks "How?" and "Why?," very physical—likes to dance, jump, skip, climb, and run.

6-10 years: Continues to be very active in play, enjoys group play but begins to choose one or two "best friends," learns to better control temper and handle frustrations, modesty increases, awareness of gender differences increases.

11-12 years: Adolescence begins. Mood swings, preoccupation with body development, argumentative, rebellious towards parents, strong need to conform with peer group, prefers to be with peers rather than with family or alone, sexual attraction is beginning.

uli can be introduced, much like infants are introduced to one new food at a time.

Note: If a biological mother is still drinking, she should not breastfeed her baby because the alcohol will be present in her breastmilk and passed on to the infant. Also, if the infant continues to have problems feeding and/or vomits often, a pediatrician should be contacted.

Making Adjustments

As children with FAS/FAE get older, they have special needs and their own unique ways of interacting and learning. Parents, teachers, and other caretakers become frustrated when they expect these children to comprehend and perform like "normal" children. One of the first things parents of children with FAS/FAE need to do is adjust their expectations to their child's abilities. One child with FAS/FAE may be good in art but unable to read beyond a third-grade level. Another child with FAS/FAE may read fairly well but not be able to remember his birth date.

A child with FAS/FAE may have several "good days or weeks" when there are no major incidents, and then do something that causes serious upheaval. To assume that a child with FAS/FAE is going to progress on an even keel may be setting parents up for bitter disappointment. Also, when this child is constantly expected to perform at a certain level that she simply isn't capable of, then her self-esteem and self-image suffer.

To avoid becoming overly frustrated with your child:

❑ Familiarize yourself with the various stages of normal child development, either by speaking with your pediatrician, taking classes, and/or reading about these topics. Then, instead of expecting your child with FAS/FAE to perform at the same level as children born without FAS/FAE, adjust your expectations according to what your child is realistically able to accomplish

❑ Focus on your child's strengths, talents and positive accomplishments (such as in art, music, individual sports), rather than his shortcomings

❑ Accept that constant repetition may be necessary. Many children with FAS/FAE are not able to retain information for very long. They need to be reminded, guided, and supervised on a daily basis

❑ Be consistent in the way you deal with your child. Set firm limits and guidelines and enforce them over and over again. Realize that if you leave your child unattended for even short periods of time, she may revert to inappropriate behaviors

❑ Use concrete examples and visual aides when attempting to teach your child something. Merely talking to him may not have much impact

❑ Use praise and positive reinforcement often

❑ Avoid setting up situations where your child will likely get into trouble or not follow through on a task you assign her. (One family sent their child to the store with money to buy a loaf of bread. Not only did the child forget what she went to the store to buy, but she didn't come home with any change. Instead, she bought $5 worth of candy. She was 13 years old)

❑ Be aware that children with FAS/FAE can easily become victims by being used by others for sex or illegal purposes. Make sure that you know where they are at all times. Remind them, daily, not to go off with strangers or allow themselves to be manipulated by others. (There is no guarantee that they will comprehend the seriousness of this, but it is still important to be consistent and repetitive. The best "insurance" is to make sure they are supervised as much as possible)

❑ Dress them in bright-colored clothing so that they can be seen by drivers and spotted in crowds to ensure their safety. You may want to put reflector tape on the clothing they wear outside at night

❑ Teach them basic social and living skills, over and over again. (See Section 2, Techniques, for more details about this)

❑ Help them learn simple money management

❑ Honor their feelings (as well as your own) and provide them with positive ways to express them

❑ Keep in mind that all children with FAS/FAE are unique individuals. Comparing them with others may cause you much frustration and disappointment. Appreciate them for who they are

The Preschool Child with FAS/FAE

A preschool setting may be the first place where a child with FAS/FAE is identified as having special needs. Compared to the other children in her class, she may exhibit developmental delays, behavioral problems, and difficulties socializing appropriately. She may also become overstimulated if there is too much noise or activity going on in the room. She needs things to be calm and orderly. Transitions should be kept to a minimum and activities introduced slowly and one at a time to her. Additional ways preschool staff can help the child with FAS/FAE include:

❑ Breaking the larger group into small groups whenever possible, so that the child will have fewer children to interact with and a greater degree of adult supervision

❑ Not expecting the child with FAS/FAE to sit and focus on one topic for any length of time, but instead allowing her to get up and move around at regular intervals (approximately every ten to fifteen minutes)

❑ Supervising the child during activity time and helping her start an activity and see it through to completion

(Often a child with FAS/FAE jumps from one activity to another before completing anything)

❑ Having an area inside or outside the classroom where the student can release anger and pent-up energy when she needs to. (See Chapter 4, pages 75–94 for examples of releasing anger/energy in appropriate ways)

❑ Always supervising her during recess and whenever there is a transition from one room to another

❑ Holding regular staff meetings to discuss her progress and updating expectations and strategies to use with her as needed

❑ Including parents in planning what is best for their child—keeping communication lines open, making appropriate referrals and documenting information that will be useful in parent/teacher conferences

❑ Assessing the child's developmental growth to determine her strengths and weaknesses and to measure her skills compared to the skills we expect children of her age to be able to master. The assessment team may include a physician, speech specialist, psychologist, physical/occupational therapist, and learning specialist

The Child with FAS/FAE in School

In order for schools to become more aware of the special needs of students with FAS/FAE and their families, educating educators is essential. Fortunately, many teachers and other school personnel have begun to request training and classes that will help them better understand the serious effects prenatal exposure to alcohol and other drugs can have on a child and how that child can remain affected for life.

If your child was born with FAS/FAE, it is important to let the school (or day care provider) know this when you enroll her. Ask if the staff is aware of what Fetal Alcohol Syndrome is. Offer to provide them with articles that will help them better understand what they are dealing with. (See articles in the back of this book that can be used for this purpose.)

You can also request that your child be evaluated by the school psychologist and/or the school's Intervention Team at various transition points as she progresses through school. For instance, evaluations are usually done in infancy, early childhood, kindergarten, elementary school, junior high (or middle) school, and high school. In some cases the evaluations may be done more frequently, and your child should be closely monitored by her school's Intervention Team every year. (See explanation of testing and school Intervention Team in Chapter 4, pages 41–59.)

By law, parents are entitled to attend meetings where the Individual Educational Plan (IEP) of their child is being discussed and their signature is required on the plan. Likewise, parents have a right to be present at Intervention Team Meetings where their child is being discussed. See page 40 for more information on the IEP.

If you meet with resistance from the first person you talk with, try to find someone else within the school or day care facility who is receptive. (Also see Dealing with Denial of FAS/FAE Within Our School System on page 62.) It is very important that the school and parents work together to meet the needs of students with FAS/FAE. Some parents have become active in their school's PTA and have educated both teachers and other parents about FAS/FAE. Together they have set up positive learning environments for students with FAS/FAE and have also banded together to send groups to legislative hearings in hopes of convincing legislators that schools need more moneys so they can better serve students with FAS/FAE. See Chapter 4 for a better understanding of students' needs and what services schools provide.

As students with FAS/FAE get older they need less emphasis on academics and more on basic living skills and vocational training. Some young adults with FAS/FAE are more capable of finishing school and holding jobs than others, but even so, they need close guidance and consistent structure, order, and routine. It is important to remember that:

> *Many adolescents and adults with FAS can be very emotionally immature*
>
> *98 percent cannot handle money wisely*
>
> *50 percent need help with basic hygiene*

There are those who would like to believe that FAS/FAE is an "affliction" that is outgrown, and that once a child reaches 18 or 21 years of age, he can function as a "normal" adult. This simply is not so. FAS/FAE is a lifelong handicap. We must accept this fact and work together to care for those who are victims of it, and educate others who can prevent it from continuing to occur.

Educating Doctors, Counselors, and Other Helping Professionals

One couple in our parent support group had their twelve-year-old son to over sixty doctors before one of the doctors mentioned the possibility of FAS/FAE. Also, many parents have said that they and their children have gone through numerous types of counseling and nothing has worked because the counselors haven't understood FAS/FAE and how to work effectively with family members.

The need for training counselors, psychologists, psychiatrists and other professionals who work with families is great. The awareness is finally growing but even so, much more has to be done. Parents banding together can do a lot to educate those who don't yet know about FAS/FAE. Public speaking, writing articles, taking literature to doctors, counselors and public health nurses can help with spreading the word. One of our parents helped organize a seminar at a local hospital where a variety of health care professionals were willing to listen to and share information with parents who attended the gathering. Radio and television talk shows also reach a wide variety of people, including those in helping professions.

The Parent Support Group

A support group for parents provides an opportunity for those raising children with FAS/FAE to meet and share their feelings and experiences, as well as any new information they may have about FAS/FAE. Parents who are in support groups of this kind say over and over again how invaluable these groups are to them because they can go there and feel totally accepted and understood. This is important—especially when so many people in our society don't yet understand FAS/FAE and aren't able to offer the parents of children with FAS/FAE the empathy and support they need and deserve.

Starting Your Own Group

The good news is that starting a group can be easy. All it takes is one person with the desire to do so. Then that person has to:

1. Decide Upon a Meeting Place.

Possible meeting places could be someone's home or office, a school, a church meeting room, a community center, the local library, or a social service agency meeting room. Often, there is no charge for the use of these facilities, especially when people know the purpose of your meeting.

2. Get the Word Out.

There are a variety of ways to advertise your meetings:

❑ Announce it in a PTA, church, community center or social service agency newsletter

❑ Distribute fliers in places where parents will see them

❏ Place an ad in a local newspaper

❏ Utilize radio and television stations that air public service announcements

❏ Contact leaders of other parent support groups and ask them to announce it to their members

❏ Organize a telephone "grapevine" to inform people of the upcoming meeting

Once the group meets for the first time, the word will spread. It only takes a few people coming together to start a group that will grow and reach many others. Then, the group needs to:

3. Establish Goals.

Some Parent Support Groups may wish to set specific goals for their group. These goals might be:

1. To create a safe environment where parents can gather to share their stories and feelings about raising children with FAS/FAE

2. To keep abreast of current research and other information about FAS/FAE such as training, community networking, legislative bills, etc.

3. To offer emotional support to each other

4. Establish Ground Rules.

It is important to take time at the first meeting to establish a group format or "ground rules." This insures safety and consistency, and is primary in building trust and rapport among group members. Some things you might want to decide upon are:

❏ Does the group want one appointed leader or will the leadership be rotated?

- ❏ Will the group be open to whoever wants to come, whenever they want to, or will it have a maximum number of members and be "closed?"
- ❏ How often will the group want to meet?
- ❏ Will there be any fees? (Especially if there is a room rental cost or any mailing expenses.)
- ❏ Does the group want to become socially and politically active? Who will represent the group?
- ❏ Will you invite guests and/or guest speakers to the meetings?
- ❏ Will you produce a newsletter or minutes of the meetings so that others who can't attend can still be part of the network?

If the group grows, you may want to break into sub-groups and meet at different locations to accommodate members who come from different areas in the community. The sub-groups may want to meet periodically as a larger group.

5. *Define Group Interaction.*

It is important to establish how members will interact with each other during the meetings. Some basic rules that help make the group successful are:

Maintain confidentiality. What is shared in the group remains in the group. Members should not tell others outside the group what someone else has said or repeat the names of members without their permission.

No interruptions. If someone is talking, it is their turn to speak and others should wait until that person is finished. You may also want to set a limit as to how long a person can talk.

Just listen. Sometimes the person speaking just needs

to talk and be listened to. No "crosstalk" or giving advice to someone during group time unless it is asked for.

Honor feelings. Let others express their feelings. Don't put down or discount what someone says. Don't "help" unless asked.

Respect meeting times. Start and end group meetings on time. As the group begins to meet regularly and grows, adjustments may be necessary simply because the group members know more about the group process and the needs of one another.

Adoptive Parents, Biological Parents

In working with both adoptive and biological parents I have found that their feelings are very similar and they have the same needs for support and guidance. Adoptive parents have told me that early on they felt responsible for their adopted child's problems. "What are we doing wrong?" they would ask themselves. When they were unable to get enough information from the adoption agency or attorney, they were discouraged and frustrated.

As our society becomes more educated about FAS/FAE, adoption agencies and attorneys should be required to provide adoptive parents and primary caretakers with a complete family history of the child's biological parents and the extent of the mother's alcohol and other chemical use during pregnancy, if there was any. Recent studies indicate that it costs $1,400,000 to support the needs of a child with FAS for her lifetime. New laws definitely need to be written that will grant financial aid to those who are willing to raise children with FAS/FAE.

At the same time, I have known a number of biological mothers who have gone into recovery, furthered their educations, and poured their energy not only into their children but into the field of alcoholism prevention and educating others about FAS/FAE. They and their families have also been instrumental in lobbying politicians for more funding and for building networking systems for FAS/FAE parent support groups.

There is much that needs to be done to prevent FAS/FAE and to help those who must already deal with it. Recovering mothers and their families, as well as adoptive parents, are strong voices in the movement that is educating others about FAS and FAE and making a difference in our society.

The Special Role of Foster Parents

Foster parents can have a significant impact on the life of a child, no matter how short the child's stay is with them. Many children with FAS/FAE have been placed in one foster home after another. They may be handicapped not only by the alcohol their mothers drank during pregnancy, but also by the trauma and upheaval they have gone through because of the environments they have been exposed to and from moving from place to place. They are often victims of physical, emotional and sexual abuse that has been going on for some time and inflicted upon them by various adults and other children. I worked with one ten-year-old child with FAS who had been in twenty-nine foster homes since birth and was totally out of control.

Foster parents need to work closely with the child's caseworker and become familiar with the history of the child with FAS/FAE that they are caring for. They should take advantage of the services available to them and the child, such as medical, dental and counseling services. It is also very important that they let their foster child's school know as much as possible about the child. Talking to his teacher(s) and school counselor is a good beginning. If the child is receiving counseling, it helps if that counselor and the school counselor consult together so that they are both working toward the same goals.

As a school counselor, I try to talk to the caseworker, foster parent, and the child's counselor on a regular basis. I then relay information about the child to his teacher and, when appropriate, the Intervention Team (see page 41). I have often counseled foster parents regarding behavior management and have also been present during parent-teacher conferences.

Children with FAS/FAE who live in foster homes need all the support they can get, as do their foster parents. Schools can provide a great deal of "daytime support" and can reinforce the support provided by outside agencies. It is also very important to follow through with Intervention Team recommendations, especially if psychological testing is recommended (See Chapter 4 about the School Intervention Team) and to keep the student's file up to date in case he moves on to another school or gets a new teacher the following year. Too often, foster children's needs are ignored because they transfer from school to school and easily "fall through the cracks." We don't have to let this continue to happen.

CHAPTER 4

Teaching the Child with FAS/FAE

It has only been recently that school districts, nationwide, have begun to understand the seriousness of Fetal Alcohol Syndrome and Fetal Alcohol Effects, and the fact that both are birth defects that are life-long and irreversible. Many teachers are asking what they can do now while their districts, communities and state funding sources determine how best to serve the academic and emotional needs of children with FAS/FAE.

Different states have specific guidelines that qualify students for special education. A recent California study indicated that it costs $14,000 per year to educate a special education student, as opposed to $4,000 per year for a student who can function well in a regular classroom. Therefore, school districts require strong evidence that students need special services.

However, teachers are beginning to realize that trying to manage just one or two children with FAS/FAE in their classrooms takes a great deal of their time and energy away from the rest of their students. Changes must be made in the way the system is presently set up. Parents, teachers and Intervention Team members are the leaders for initiating the changes needed.

The Optimum School Environment

Children with FAS/FAE function best when there is *structure, order,* and *routine.* In addition to teaching them academics, we must also teach them basic living skills, social skills, and anger management. Their inability to behave and perform like other children is not their fault. Too often they are punished, teased, humiliated, and rejected because they can not "keep up" with their classmates. They are accused of being "lazy," "troublemakers," "spaced-out," and/or "out to purposely get" their teachers and other students. The reality is that they have a birth defect that causes them to think, act, and relate differently than the other students. Now that they are in school, they deserve to learn as much as they are capable of learning in a safe, healthy, caring environment.

At this time, we know that most students with FAS/FAE function best when:

❑ The classroom is small (eight to ten students)

❑ It is self-contained

❑ There is minimal change

❑ Stimulation is kept at a minimum

❑ Rules and guidelines are clear and consistent

❑ Expectations are realistic

❑ There is as much one-to-one attention and supervision as possible (three adults to eight students is recommended)

❑ Positive reinforcement is used

❑ Curriculums allow the student to be successful the majority of the time

❑ Students' feelings are acknowledged and there is a plan for them to be expressed in appropriate ways

❑ Communication between teachers and parents is clear and open

It is often difficult for students with FAS/FAE to:

❑ Stay on task

❑ Refrain from being in constant motion

❑ Refrain from being disruptive

❑ Work independently for long periods of time

❑ Distinguish right from wrong/learn from their mistakes

❑ Use good judgment

❑ Control their impulses

❑ Retain what they learn from one day to the next

A Word of Caution

Before we assume that a child is either FAS or FAE, it is important to keep in mind that many of their characteristics may be similar to those found in students with Attention Deficit Disorder or other behavior disorders. Characteristics shared may be:

Hyperactivity

Impulsivity

Inability to stay on task or complete tasks

Being disruptive

Poor social skills

Demanding lots of attention

Disregard for rules and authority

Learning disabilities

In some school districts, nurses are being trained to do initial screenings of students suspected to have FAS or FAE. If it seems fairly certain that the child has FAS or FAE, then that child needs to be staffed by the Intervention Team and a recommendation needs to be made to the parents that the child be diagnosed by a trained physician, as explained in Chapter 1.

The school psychologist will decide which academic and psychological tests to administer and discuss this with the Intervention Team. It is important to remember that most testing situations provide the student with FAS/FAE with the type of environment they function best in—a quiet place with few distractions and one-on-one supervision.

When Testing Is Done and Scores Are High, Then What?

Even when some children are diagnosed with FAS or FAE, they can still score high on academic tests—too high, in fact, to permit them to be in special education classrooms. When a student's academic progress is too high for Special Education placement, another way to make him eligible is to cite his behavior as something that interferes with his learning.

If the student does score high academically, then it may be advised that the classroom teacher and other staff members provide anecdotal records of the child's behavior, over a specific period of time. If behaviors are consistently inappropriate and interfere with the student's ability to learn, then he may be eligible for special education because of a Behavior Disorder.

The Individualized Education Plan (IEP)

The Individualized Education Plan is required for Special Education students. IEP forms are generally filled out in the fall and then again in the spring, to measure the student's progress and to determine where the student should be placed next year. Parents are asked to participate in the

IEP conference, and the IEP form must be signed by one of the parents.

The School Intervention Team

Developing an IEP for a student with FAS/FAE requires the working together of a team of staff members who fully understand FAS/FAE. Typically, intervention teams are made up of the school's:

Principal

Psychologist

Nurse

Counselor and / or social worker

Classroom teacher of the student

Basic skills teacher

Special education and / or resource room teacher

Others: Physical education teacher, instructional aide, occupational therapist, family support workers, etc.

Goals of the Intervention Team

The goals of the Intervention Team should be:

❏ To determine whether or not the student should be made a Focus of Concern based on academic and/or behavior performance

❏ To recommend psychological testing when appropriate

❏ To discuss strategies that will provide the student with a safe, positive atmosphere and environment for learning

❏ To plan a curriculum that includes teaching basic living skills, social skills and anger management

INDIVIDUALIZED EDUCATION PROGRAM
ELEMENTARY LEVEL

Student's Name	Soc. Sec. #	Student No.	Birthdate	H.C.	Grade	School Year	IEP Type
			9/21/82	HI	4	1992–93	Continuing

Parent/Guardian	Street Address	City	Zip	Phone

Is a Surrogate Parent needed?	Ethnic Group	Home School	Service School	IEP Date	Review Date
No	W			1/19/92	11/20/93

Reading

Stanford Diagnostic Reading Test

Administration Date	11/91	11/92
Test Level	Red	Green
Auditory Discrimination	1.0	5.3
Phonetic Analysis	1.9	NA
Structural Analysis	NA	3.4
Auditory Vocabulary	2.5	3.8
Word Reading	2.4	NA
Reading Comprehension	3.2	NA
Literal Comprehension	NA	3.2
Inferential Comprehension	NA	3.2
Comprehension Total	2.4	3.6

Woodcock-Johnson - Revised

Administration Date	
Basic Reading Skills	
Reading Comprehension	

Reading Program: Reading Mastery
Instructional level: II

Math Program: Addison-Wesley
Instructional level: 3rd/4th (mod)

Mathematics

Stanford Diagnostic Arithmetic Test

	10/91	10/92
	Red	Green
Number Systems/Numerat	1.9	3.2
Computation	1.5	3.8
Applications	1.9	3.1
Total	1.9	3.3

Woodcock-Johnson - Revised

Administration Date	
Math Calculation	
Math Applied Problems	

Written Language

Test of Written Spelling

	10/91	10/92
Administration Date		
Spelling Achievement	2.4	2.9

Woodcock-Johnson - Revised

Administration Date	
Broad Written Language	

Language Program: Spelling
Instructional level: B

Current Levels of Performance/Goals

Narrative comments need to address the child's current functioning in physical, adjustment, and academic areas, including mainstreamed contact.

PHYSICAL: _____ is a 10 year old male in 4th grade. _____ has been diagnosed with Fetal Alcohol Syndrome. Hearing is within normal limits. Vision is also within normal limits with his glasses. Stature is small for his age. There are no other gross motor concerns at this time. Fine motor skills are below grade level, but _____ has learned to cope very well. His handwriting is legible although his letters are segmented and he does not retrace on all letters. Fine motor skills will be addressed informally in the CLC.

SCHOOL DISTRICT
INDIVIDUALIZED EDUCATION PROGRAM

Student's Name	Student No.	Birthdate	School Year	IEP Type
		9/21/82	1992–93	Continuing

Current Levels of Performance Goals

*Narrative comments need to address the child's current functioning in **physical**, **adjustment**, and **academic** areas, including **mainstreamed contact**.*

ADJUSTMENT: _____ did not have to adjust to many new things this year. He came back to school in August ready to learn and move forward. His behavior is fairly predictable, but not consistent. _____ needs to feel structure, see structure, and be structured. He has the most difficulty in settings that are free, such as recess, lunch, and choice time. He tends to become silly, busy, and sometimes makes inappropriate (but not severe) choices. (Spitting, running on the sidewalk, jumping over chairs . . .) Stubbornness is still an issue with _____. It seems to be a fundamental part of his personality. He can also be argumentative. Logic and explanation don't work well in these situations. Very often _____ cannot verbalize his frustrations. He responds to distractions and redirection of his attention. At this point, time-outs or further consequences have not been necessary. However, they are in place— _____ is aware of them, and they can be used if behavior escalates. The majority of the time, _____ is a treat to have. He has wonderful ideas to share. He is kind to his peers. He is well liked by others. And _____ does try very hard to please his teachers.

ACADEMICS: _____ has made significant gains over the past year in reading and in math. Test scores have increased by over a full year. He is currently working in Reading Mastery II and will soon move to level III. Comprehension questions are more difficult for _____ in that he has a hard time pulling together all the parts to get the big idea. In math, _____ is working in the Addison-Wesley 3rd grade math book. Concepts that were fuzzy to him last year, are now clearer. He needs continued practice with the application level of math—telling time, counting money, grocery store math, etc. Written language is _____ weakest area. He has a wonderful imagination, but has difficulty with the process of getting those thoughts down correctly on paper. All three of these areas will be addressed in this IEP as well as behavior.

MAINSTREAM CONTACT: _____ is mainstreamed into a regular 4th grade class for PE, Music, recesses and lunch. His other teachers report that he can be very easily distracted and sometimes exhibits inappropriate behaviors. (See behavioral objectives.)

43

SCHOOL DISTRICT
INDIVIDUALIZED EDUCATION PROGRAM

Student's Name	Student No.	Birthdate	School Year	IEP Type
		9/21/82	1992–93	Continuing

Least Restrictive Placement

The program outlined below, including any identified related services, is considered to be the least restrictive program in which this student's needs can be met at this time.

Program Summary

Classroom Programs

	Est Min/Week	Est Start
Regular Education	375–400	11/92
Special Education		
specially designed instruction	895–920	11/92
general education components	535	11/92

P.E. Programs

Regular P.E.	70	11/92
Adjusted P.E.	0	

Vocational Programs

Regular vocational education program (incl. NEVAC)	0	
Special Education pre-vocational/vocational program	0	

Related Services (Requires goals and objectives) | IUs/yr

Communication Therapy	0
Occupational Therapy	0
Physical Therapy	0
Other	0

Each I.U. (Intervention Unit) equals one 10-minute time block.

Extended School Year (ESY) Services:
This student is NOT ELIGIBLE

Transition Plan Included? _____

I.E.P. Committee

Signatures:

_____	_____
Signature	Position
_____	_____
Signature	Position

Placement Options

Continue Regular Program	Reject
Itinerant Support	Reject
Learning Center Classes	Reject

	Elem:	Reading: ___	Math: ___	Wr. Lang: ___	Social: ___	St. Sk.: ___	Accept
	Sec:	L.A.: ___	Math: ___	Soc. Studies: ___		Study Skills: ___	Reject

Contained Learning Center	Reject
Outside Agency or Other District	
Other	

☐ My rights and responsibilities have been explained to me in a manner which I fully understand, and I have received a copy of the Procedural Safeguards document.

☐ I have had the opportunity to participate in the development of this individualized Education Plan, and I approve of the annual goals, short-term objectives, and the program placement as stated above.

☐ I concur with the other members of this IEP committee that the program/placement outlined above is the Least Restrictive Placement at this time.

☐ Parent   ☐ Guardian   ☐ Adult Student
☐ Surrogate Parent   ☐ Adult Acting in Role of Parent

_____	_____
	Date
District Representative	Date

_____	_____
Signature	Position
Signature	Position

44

SCHOOL DISTRICT
INDIVIDUALIZED EDUCATION PROGRAM

Student's Name	Student No.	Birthdate 9/21/82	School Year 1992–93	IEP Type Continuing

Annual Goal: _____ will increase his reading skills from 3.6 to 4.6 by 11/93 as measured by the Stanford Diagnostic Reading Test.

Anticipated Start Date	Anticipated End Date	Short Term Objectives	Comments	Date Met
11/92	11/93	Given a list of sight words from the Reading Mastery II and III Series, read them with 100% accuracy in 4 out of 5 trials as measured by performance and teacher data by 11/93.		
11/92	11/93	Given the Reading Mastery lesson, maintain an 80% average or better on daily skill and comprehension work as measured by written work by 11/93.		
11/92	11/93	Given the Multiple Skills Series, maintain an 80% average or better on written comprehension questions as measured by daily work by 11/93.		

SCHOOL DISTRICT
INDIVIDUALIZED EDUCATION PROGRAM

Student's Name		Student No.		Birthdate 9/21/82	School Year 1992–93	IEP Type Continuing

Annual Goal: _____ will increase spelling skills from 2.9 to 3.9 by 11/93 as measured by the Test of Written Spelling.
(2)

Anticipated Start Date	Anticipated End Date	Short Term Objectives	Comments	Date Met
11/92	11/93	Given the Spelling Mastery objectives for level B, pass each objective with 80% accuracy or better as measured by test data through 11/93.		
11/92	11/93	Given weekly spelling tests, maintain an 80% average or better as measured by test data through 11/93.		
11/92	3/93	Given oral dictation, write a 5+ word sentence with correct punctuation with 100% accuracy as measured by performance and teacher data by 3/93.		
2/93	11/93	Given oral dictation, write a 5+ word sentence with correct spelling, punctuation and capitalization with 90% accuracy or better as measured by performance and teacher data by 11/93.		
11/92	3/93	Given a topic, write 3+ complete sentences with 80% accuracy or better as measured by performance and teacher data by 3/93.		
2/93	11/93	Given a topic, write 3+ complete sentences with appropriate capitalization and punctuation with 90% accuracy or better as measured by performance and teacher data by 11/93.		

46

SCHOOL DISTRICT
INDIVIDUALIZED EDUCATION PROGRAM

Student's Name	Student No.	Birthdate	School Year	IEP Type
		9/21/82	1992–93	Continuing

Annual Goal: _____
(3) will increase math skills from 3.3 to 4.3 by 11/1/93 as measured by the Stanford Diagnostic Math Test.

Anticipated Start Date	Anticipated End Date	Short Term Objectives	Comments	Date Met
11/92	1/93	Given 10 more addition problems (3 and 4 digit, plus 1, 2, 3 and 4 digit, carrying once to the ten's column), solve with 80% accuracy or better as measured by ICSP.		
11/92	1/93	Given 10 or more addition problems (2, 3, and 4 digit, plus 2, 3 and 4 digit, carrying once to the hundreds column), solve with 80% accuracy or better as measured by ICSP.		
12/92	6/93	Given 10 or more subtraction problems (2 and 3 digit, minus 1, 2, and 3 digit, borrowing from the tens), solve with 80% accuracy or better as measured by ICSP.		
12/92	6/93	Given ten or more subtraction problems (3 digit, minus 2, and 3 digit, borrowing from the hundreds), solve with 80% accuracy or better as measured by ICSP.		
3/93	11/93	Given 10 or more subtraction problems (3 digit, minus 2, and 3 digit, borrowing from the tens and hundreds), solve with 80% accuracy or better as measured by ICSP.		
1/93	6/93	Given 10 mixed addition and subtraction problems that require regrouping, solve with 90% accuracy or better as measured by performance on written work and teacher data by 6/93.		
11/92	11/93	Given a clock, tell time to 5 minute intervals with 100% accuracy as measured by teacher evaluation by 11/93.		
12/92	3/93	Given various coins, count their value with 100% accuracy as measured by teacher evaluation by 3/93.		

SCHOOL DISTRICT
INDIVIDUALIZED EDUCATION PROGRAM

Student's Name		Student No.	Birthdate 9/21/82	School Year 1992–93	IEP Type Continuing

Annual Goal: _____ will increase appropriate behaviors to match those of his same-aged peers as measured by teacher observations by 11/93.
(4)

Anticipated Start Date	Anticipated End Date	Short Term Objectives	Comments	Date Met
11/92	3/93	Given an independent work period, increase time on task from 40% to 60% or better as measured by teacher observation by 3/93.		
3/93	6/93	Given an independent work period, increase time on task from 60% to 80% or better as measured by teacher observation by 6/93.		
11/92	6/93	Given a large group discussion, increase attending and active participation from 60% to 90% or better as measured by teacher observation by 6/93.		
11/92	11/93	Given a freetime period, initiate play and/or conversation with a peer on 5 out of 5 days or more as measured by teacher observation by 11/93.		
11/92	11/93	Given the playground setting, demonstrate appropriate interaction with peers 90% of the time as measured by teacher data by 11/93.		
11/92	11/93	Given oral directions of 2 to 3 parts, follow the directions with 100% accuracy or better as measured by teacher observation by 11/93.		
11/92	11/93	Given oral directions, follow the directions without arguing or negative comments 80% of the time or better as measured by teacher observation by 11/93.		
11/92	6/93	Given a playground and school grounds setting, verbalize to a peer or adult the emotion felt in a situation and participate in problem solving before reacting physically or verbally 80% of the time or better as measured by teacher data by 6/93.		

48

❏ To focus on the strengths of the student so that she feels some degree of success each day

❏ To determine ways to monitor the student's behavior so that she isn't a threat to herself, or others

❏ To keep communication open with parents, paying close attention to the initial contact with the parent following the Intervention Team meeting

To be aware of cultural diversity

To understand the feelings/stigma associated with alcoholism

To provide referral sources to parents

❏ To be open to ongoing research, updates about FAS/FAE

❏ To network with other community resources

❏ To provide support for each other

It is important that the school acknowledges the value of informed parents and strives to work as a team with them. Many parents who have children with FAS/FAE are the best resources for helping school personnel understand what their children need in school, what their strengths are, how to deal with certain behaviors, what has and hasn't worked with their children in the past, etc.

The Meeting Format

Most Intervention Teams meet once per week and spend thirty to forty-five minutes staffing two individual students. The classroom teacher is present and usually has been the one to request the staffing. (At the school where I work, the teacher is the one who fills out the initial form to request the staffing.)

It is also helpful if the teacher from the year before is there, or the current teacher has at least been able to talk to that teacher (if the student's former school is within the district or community). The current teacher also brings the file of the student to the meeting.

STAFFING SUMMARY

Student_____ Grade_____ Date_____

Requested by_____ Teacher_____

A. Brief review of concern(s)—by referral source

B. Background information:
   1. *Student's strengths*
   2. *Student's weaknesses*
   3. *Test results / health information / parent information*
   4. *Home environment / CEE factors*

C. Input from Team Members

D. Intervention strategies and Implementation
   1. *Brainstorming*
   2. *Interventions*

Intervention/ objectives	Responsible staff member	By what date
A.		
B.		
C.		

E. Will child be made a Focus of Concern (FOC)?_____
   <u>Note</u>: Decision to file a FOC is made provided *FOC Criteria* have been met.

F. Follow-up staffing date (normally 4–6 weeks)_____
   1. *Review of interventions and progress*
   2. *Closure or additional action needed*

CONFIDENTIAL **DATE:**_____

CHILD STUDY TEAM
(Request for Staffing—Referral Information)

Student_____ Grade_____ Birthdate_____

Requested by_____(brings student file)

Teacher_____Reading Teacher_____

Academic/Behavioral Concerns_____
_____
_____

Other Observations_____
_____

Interventions Employed to Date:

1. _____

2. _____

3. _____

Should last year's teacher attend?___(If so, name_____)

COMPLETE TOP PORTION AND RETURN TO RESOURCE TEACHER

- -

The following people should attend:

_____Principal _____Counselor _____CH.I Teacher

_____Psychologist _____Nurse _____P.E. Teacher

_____Resource Teacher _____CDS Others:_____

Staffing date and time:_____

Please come prepared to contribute your perspective of the problem and include data from tests, class work, etc.

Intervention Team members go over the file together and, if they know the student, each member comments on what they have observed about her. Occasionally, the parent(s) will be present, especially if they have been the ones to request the staffing. During the staffing, team members write out a specific plan that identifies strategies the classroom teacher (and other staff members who work with the student) will use. It is also decided when there will be a follow-up on the student (generally within two to three weeks) to see how the strategies are working. It may be recommended that the parent(s) attend the follow-up session or that a meeting between the principal, the parent(s) and team members be set up so that the parent understands the concerns of the team.

Contacting the Parent

Determining who will be the staff person to contact the parent about suspected FAS/FAE and permission to test the student is something that has to be carefully considered. It is good to keep in mind that there is much guilt and shame associated with the disease of alcoholism. Birth mothers who are still drinking may be too involved with their alcoholism to attend to their children's needs, including their educational needs. Birth mothers who are in recovery may find it difficult to face the fact that their child has been so greatly affected by their drinking during pregnancy. Even adoptive parents sometimes have a hard time admitting that anything is wrong with their child because they perceive it as a reflection of their parenting skills and/or the reality of something being wrong with their child is too overwhelming to them.

If there has been a rapport established previously between the parent and an Intervention Team member, then this member is probably the one who should make the initial contact, even if it is simply to introduce another team member such as the nurse, psychologist, social worker, or counselor who can discuss with the parent in more detail the concerns of the Intervention Team and why psychological testing has been recommended.

It is good to determine, as a team, where the meeting with the parents should take place. Should it be held at school? If so, where? In the classroom (usually before or after school), or in the office of the counselor, psychologist, nurse, principal, or other involved staff member? In instances where the parents aren't able to get to the school, a home visit may be appropriate. Many schools have social workers and/or family support workers who have already been to the home and have a good relationship with the parent.

During the meeting with the parent, it is important to find out as much as possible about the mother's pregnancy. Questions to ask might include:

❑ Tell me about your pregnancy.

❑ Were there any complications?

❑ What type of prenatal medical care were you receiving?

❑ How would you describe your nutrition during pregnancy?

❑ What type of rest were you getting?

❑ How would you describe your emotional state during your pregnancy?

❑ Were there any traumas?

❑ What over-the-counter drugs, if any, did you use during pregnancy?

❑ What is your family's medical history?

❑ Are there medical problems that your child may be affected by?

❑ How would you describe the use of drugs or alcohol in your family?

❑ What were *your* drinking patterns during pregnancy?

If the parent becomes defensive, immediately slow down and remind yourself that your conversation will only go as far as the parent is ready for it to go. Perhaps you'll make more progress next time or someone else on staff will be the one to hear additional information. School nurses have reported that parents are sometimes more open in responding to them because their questions are perceived as being part of a normal medical intake rather than information that may be used against them or their children.

When the parent you are talking to is the father, reword your questions accordingly. For instance, you may say:

❑ Tell me what you remember about your wife's pregnancy. (And follow up with the same questions you would ask the birth mother about her pregnancy.)

❑ What is your family's medical history?

❑ How would you describe the use of drugs or alcohol in your family?

❑ What recollection do you have of your wife's drinking patterns during the pregnancy?

When talking with adoptive parents, ask them how much they know about the birth mother's family history, her pregnancy, and her drinking and other drug patterns. If they don't know about these things, encourage them to try to find out about them, if possible.

Discipline

It is also important to consider what kind of living environment the child has come from or is currently in. Statistics show that children with FAS/FAE often come from backgrounds where they have been or are being abused. As you talk to parents, ask them about their methods of discipline and what they have found works and doesn't work with their child.

It may benefit parents to know that there are three main types of discipline: Authoritarian, Permissive, and Authoritative.

❑ Authoritarian:

High in control (rigid, inflexible)

Low in communication skills

Expectations are too high

Low in warmth and positive reinforcement

❑ Permissive:

Too low in control

High in communication

Expectations are too low

High in warmth

❑ Authoritative:

High in control (but fair)

High in communication

Expectations are appropriate

High in warmth and positive reinforcement

Often in dysfunctional families, one parent is authoritarian and the other parent is permissive. It is very important that discipline be consistent and congruent at home, at school, and in treatment and therapeutic settings. The authoritative model is the one that works best. Children need to know who is in charge but also want that person to be fair. Clear communication is important, and expectations should match what the child is capable of. Warmth and positive reinforcement are much better motivators than threats and punishments.

Some methods of positive discipline include:

❑ Practicing mutual respect and regard

❑ Avoiding power struggles

❑ Setting firm limits

❑ Being consistent (and united when working in a team)

❑ Acknowledging the feelings associated with the behavior

❑ When appropriate, giving children input into the plan

❑ Avoiding physical punishment because violence breeds violence

It helps if the parents and the classroom teacher can decide upon definite strategies that will be carried out at school and at home, so that discipline is similar and consistent. Some teachers and parents have agreed upon "daily reports" going home with the child or discussions over the telephone between the teacher and the parents. Giving rewards for positive behavior and having consequences for negative behavior is a method most often used. Some rewards for positive behavior might be: points, stickers, and chips that earn the student a food treat, a movie, a trip to the park, a toy under $5, etc. Consequences for negative behavior might include: no TV for a specific amount of time, no playing video games, going to bed early, no dessert for a week, etc.

Parents and teachers may be tempted to restrict the child from playing outside as a consequence for negative behavior, but because physical exercise helps with hyperactivity, the lack of it may make matters even worse. It is better to choose other types of consequences.

Example of Daily Report:

	Good	Average	Hard Day	Comments
Homework				
Behavior				
Class Assignments				
Energy Level				

Being Sensitive to Cultural Values and Beliefs

In dealing with parents you must also be very aware and respectful of the diversity of cultures our schools now serve. When preparing to contact a parent whose ethnic background is different from your own, it would be wise to first consult with a person of the parent's same ethnic background, so that you can gain a better understanding of the culture, how best to communicate with the parent during the meeting, and how the values, beliefs, and ways of doing things in that culture may be different from your own. One of our immediate goals should be to create strong networks within our communities that are multicultural and interdisciplinary, whose participants are well-trained in FAS/FAE. These networks can work in tandem with schools, exchanging information and services and serving as a support and referral system for families affected by FAS/FAE.

When parents and schools cooperate with each other, much good can come out of the relationship. Not only will some of the frustration that is so often associated with trying to teach a child with FAS/FAE be reduced, but the student also benefits from the efforts of his teachers and parents to create a positive learning environment for him.

When Parents Won't Cooperate

As mentioned before, not all parents are willing to cooperate with school staff. Teachers and other school personnel are sometimes blamed for the student's misbehavior or failure to do well academically. Or, the parents deny, minimize or rationalize the concerns that school staff may have. Some parents agree that there are problems, but fail to seek outside help for their child or to follow through with suggestions made by school staff that might help the student.

This can be very frustrating, to say the least. When there is little or no cooperation from the parent, then it is up to the principal and members of the Intervention Team to consider what other options are available. Some of the options may include:

❑ Discussing the kinds of special services the student can receive without parental consent (for instance, a tutor or aide working one-on-one with the child in the classroom)

❑ Determining ways to monitor the student more closely to eliminate possible behavior problems (constant supervision during recess, in the lunchroom, to and from various classes, etc.)

❑ Documenting all incidents that are of concern, including date, time, description of the incident and parties involved

❑ Scheduling regular staffings on the child so that school personnel can update information and strategies

❑ Drawing up a written contract between the student and appropriate staff (his teacher, counselor or the principal) so that the student and the parents have a written document stating the expectations of the school. Ask that this contract be signed by both the student and his parents. (Contracts are usually used with students who are eight years old and older. Contracts for younger children should be primarily between parents and school staff)

In some cases, especially when a student is being harmful to himself or others or is destroying the property of the school or others, then he will have to be suspended. Sometimes a series of suspensions makes parents realize that their child really does need help and they will take action to get that help for him and/or agree to cooperate more with the school. Also see Strategies for Inside and Outside the Classroom on page 60.

Example of Written Contract Between Student and Teacher

CONTRACT

March 4, 199_

I _____ agree to the following contract between me and my teacher to help me improve my behavior and study habits in school.

1. When I feel restless I will let my teacher know and then spend time at my special desk until I can calm down.

2. When I feel angry I will tell my teacher and we will decide how much time I need and where I will go to get my anger out in a safe way.

3. On days that I don't bring my homework or when I need help with an assignment, I will give up part of my recess time so that I can stay in and get my work done. I understand that I may have to stay after school if it doesn't get completed. (If so, my parents will be called when I have to stay after school so they won't worry about where I am.)

4. When there are field trips, I understand that one of my parents will have to come along so that I can get the attention I need and stay safe.

5. If I have a bad day I know that my teacher will have to let my parents know and that I will not get to watch T.V. or play with my video games that night. When I have a good day, I will get a sticker. When I earn 5 stickers, my teacher will let me choose a prize from her prize box.

     Signed   Student

                           Teacher

                           Parent

Mainstreaming Versus the Self-Contained Classroom

The latest philosophy in education is to mainstream as many special needs children as possible. Unfortunately, many students with FAS/FAE tend to have problems learning and behaving when they are placed in regular classrooms. One main reason for this is that their ability to filter too much stimulation is very limited. The noise, visual images, and energy that is generated by a roomful of students can become too much for them. As a mother of a child with FAS described it,

> When my son is put into a busy classroom with twenty-seven other students, it can be as unnerving for him as it would be for you or me to be stuck in the middle of a shopping mall with a migraine headache, on an exceptionally busy day.

It isn't fair to the child with FAS/FAE to be expected to function in an environment that is too stimulating and where there may be several transitions to other classes during the day. Neither is it fair to the teacher and the other students. Until the educational system accepts that many students with FAS/FAE should not be mainstreamed, there are several things teachers can do both inside and outside their classrooms to make things more manageable for their students with FAS/FAE and for themselves.

Strategies for Inside and Outside the Classroom

It is essential that you have strategies to use for students with FAS/FAE both inside and outside the classroom, and that all school staff know what these strategies are. Sometimes, two teachers may have an agreement to assist each other when extra attention must be given to a student with FAS/FAE. For instance, if the child just needs a short break from the routine of the classroom, his teacher may send him across the hall to the other teacher's room, with a note requesting a book or some other item. This enables the student to move around and also makes him feel important. (The student may have to be watched as he crosses the hall. This will depend on his ability to stay on task.) The same teachers may also have an understanding that one will check on the other's classroom if a student with FAS/FAE needs to be escorted to another part of the building.

Other strategies for inside and outside the classroom may include:

Inside the Classroom

❏ Where can the child sit so that he will be able to focus better and be the least disruptive? Some teachers use carrels around the student's desk to help block out too much stimulation. Other teachers have a desk located in the back or side of the room for the student to go to. It is important that whatever the set-up is, it should not be perceived by the student as punitive.

❏ What is the child's learning style? Is he visual, auditory, kinesthetic?

❏ What can the teacher realistically expect from the student academically? (If the child has trouble keeping up with the others in his class, assignments may have to be shortened or changed so that he has a better chance of being successful.)

❏ How can the teacher build on the student's strengths?

❏ Who is available to work one-on-one with the child (an aide, intern, parent or other volunteers)?

❏ What types of discipline work or don't work?

❏ What strategies should be used if the child has an outburst in class? For example, does the teacher leave his class to deal with the child one-on-one in private? Or, should the student be sent to the counselor, principal, or designated other?

Outside the Classroom

❑ What is the plan for recess? Does the child have adequate supervision?

❑ Who will supervise during lunch time?

❑ Who will accompany the child when the classroom is not self-contained and students go elsewhere for reading, math, music, etc.? Will it be an adult or another student from the room?

❑ Will the child be allowed to go on field trips? If so, who will supervise the child one-on-one? If not, where will he go within the school?

These are just some of the things to consider. Since all children are so unique, there may be other needs (not listed here) that they will have. These too, will have to be discussed. Implementing certain strategies for a student with FAS/FAE will have to be done on a trial-and-error basis. Ultimately, the principal has to make the final decision as to how much the school can do for the student without parent cooperation.

Working with a child who has FAS/FAE can be an ongoing challenge. One person cannot "do it all." The team approach is best and including parents, especially when they are cooperative, can help insure that the student's educational, social and emotional needs are met. Also, by enlisting the help of outside agencies and professionals for training, consultation and referral, a stronger network is built to support the schools and the families they serve.

Dealing with Denial of FAS/FAE Within Our School Systems

Occasionally a teacher or parent will approach me and ask how they can break through the denial in their school that FAS/FAE exists. Even though the research has been going on for years, the reality of FAS/FAE has only recently come to the attention of many in our society. We have to be patient with those who are still finding it difficult to accept. I encourage teachers to seek out other teachers and staff in their schools who are at least open to learning more about this birth defect. With parents, I suggest the same thing. They can share information and try some of the strategies and techniques outlined in this handbook. They can request trainings on the topic and possibly get the support of the PTA. Because this problem is growing, sooner or later those who want to ignore it won't be able to do so any longer, especially if parents and teachers continue to voice their needs and join together to get these needs met.

A Summary of What Schools Can Do for Their Students with FAS/FAE

1. Educators need to become educated about FAS/FAE, keeping in mind that parental input can often be just as valuable as classes and workshops on this topic

2. Schools need to set up Screening and Intervention Teams to deal with the needs of students with FAS/FAE

3. Teachers need assistance in the classroom when they have students with FAS/FAE. This assistance may come from student teachers, aides, parent volunteers, tutors, basic skills teachers, instructional assistants, etc.

4. In addition to academics, students with FAS/FAE need to be taught basic living skills, social skills and in the upper grades, vocational skills. Anger management is also recommended for those with anger problems

5. Students with FAS/FAE benefit from smaller classrooms, minimal change, constant supervision, one-on-one attention, and consistent positive reinforcement

6. Schools can play a key role in networking with other community agencies and professionals to build pro-

grams and provide counseling for students with FAS/FAE and their families

7. Schools provide an excellent environment for teaching prevention. FAS and FAE are birth defects that are totally preventable

8. School personnel can be powerful lobbyists for more funding for school programs tailored for students with FAS/FAE, and for re-writing laws that determine who is eligible for special services

Section *II*

Techniques for Working with Children, Adolescents, and Adults with FAS/FAE

*T*echniques that are most successful with children with FAS/FAE need to be visual, concrete, and repeated often. Because it is not easy for these children to retain information, it is important that you keep your messages to them simple and to-the-point. Also, even though most children with FAS/FAE are very verbal, they don't always get the connection between words and concepts. Instead, they are more likely to understand what they can see and experience hands-on.

We know that what children with FAS/FAE appear to understand today may have to be re-taught tomorrow. We also know that they become easily frustrated, have low impulse control, often use poor judgment and are not always able to distinguish right from wrong.

Many of the techniques introduced in this section were created to help children with FAS/FAE modify their behaviors and learn to express their feelings and emotions in positive ways. Teaching them requires patience, and the belief that children with FAS/FAE deserve to be empowered on a

65

daily basis. The following techniques do empower and build self-esteem, and they also provide the children with simple, visual images that have a lasting impact.

Also, even though these techniques may seem rather juvenile, they work with older children just as they do with younger ones. Adolescents and adults with FAS/FAE may have adult-sized bodies, but emotionally they can be quite young and relate well to examples geared for younger children.

These techniques have also proven successful with children who have behavior problems.

CHAPTER 5

*Techniques for
Helping Children
Through Adults*

Better Understanding the Child

Techniques:

❑ Who Listens to You the Best?

❑ Getting in Touch with Feelings

❑ The Target

❑ The Time Line

❑ The Thermometer

❑ The Body Picture

There can be many reasons why children with FAS/FAE act the way they do. Some are directly associated with their being FAS/FAE. Others are due to what they have experienced while growing up. These techniques will help you better understand the needs of children with FAS/FAE, what causes some of their behaviors, and which issues need to be addressed with them and their families.

Who Listens to You the Best?

Appropriate for Ages: 4 to Adult.

Materials Needed: Paper and colored pens or crayons.

Goal: To help child identify who listens to him.

Follow-up: Discuss the child's drawings with him and find out why he has made the choices he has and how these individuals demonstrate good listening skills.

Setting: One-on-one.

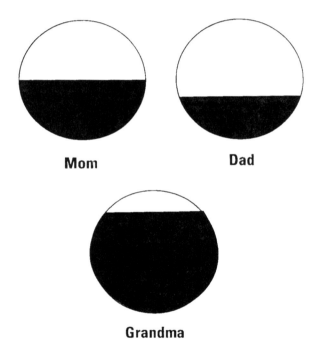

Mom   **Dad**

Grandma

Ask the child to name the people in his life that he talks to the most (family members, teachers, babysitters, etc.). Then draw a circle for each of these people. Instruct the child to fill in each circle, according to how well that person listens. (A circle completely filled in would indicate a good listener, a circle only half filled in would indicate a so-

so listener, etc. You may have to demonstrate one circle for the child so that the directions are clear.)

Once the circles are drawn in, talk to the child about each person, how they listen to him, what more he needs from them, and how he can practice good listening skills. When children report that lots of yelling occurs at home and in the classroom, this exercise can also be used to indicate who does the yelling and how much.

Getting in Touch with Feelings

Appropriate for Ages: 3 through 8.

Materials Needed: Toy or unloaded camera, mirror, tape recorder.

Goal: To familiarize child with her feelings and expression of them.

Follow-up: To talk about how the exercise felt and reinforce that feelings are okay.

Setting: One-on-one or in group.

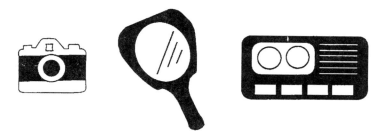

Tell the child that you are going to pretend that you are taking a picture of her. Ask her to make her most angry face for you. When she does so, show her what she looks like in the mirror. Then ask her to make her angriest sounds into the tape recorder. Replay her sounds for her. Finally, ask the child how her body feels when she is angry and where the feelings are the strongest. (One child may say she feels like she has a rock in her stomach, another child may describe a strong pressure in his chest, etc.) Repeat this same procedure using sadness, fear, and happiness as feelings to describe.

The Target

Appropriate for Ages: 6 through 12.

Materials Needed: Sheet of paper, colored pens.

Goal: To make a "map" of the child's life experience.

Follow-up: To gain a better understanding of events that have contributed to the child's view of life and patterns of behavior.

Setting: This is a one-on-one exercise, however, additional input from the parent or caregiver may be helpful.

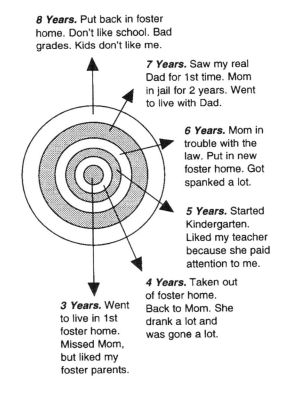

8 Years. Put back in foster home. Don't like school. Bad grades. Kids don't like me.

7 Years. Saw my real Dad for 1st time. Mom in jail for 2 years. Went to live with Dad.

6 Years. Mom in trouble with the law. Put in new foster home. Got spanked a lot.

5 Years. Started Kindergarten. Liked my teacher because she paid attention to me.

4 Years. Taken out of foster home. Back to Mom. She drank a lot and was gone a lot.

3 Years. Went to live in 1st foster home. Missed Mom, but liked my foster parents.

With younger children the target works best because it is a visual thing they can relate to. Take a piece of paper and fold it in half so that the target drawing can go on one side and ages and corresponding events can go on the other. The center (or bull's-eye) of the target is the starting point for recording the earliest events the child can remember. Each successive circle around the bull's-eye represents another year of the child's life. Make the circles different colors. Each time you draw a new circle, draw an arrow of the same color from that circle to the other side of the paper. Then record the age and the events associated with that circle. The concept is the same that is used with older children in the Time Line. It is a way of gathering information and putting the facts down on paper in a creative way.

The Time Line

Appropriate for Ages: 13 to adult.

Materials Needed: Large sheet of paper (such as butcher paper) and colored pens.

Goal: To make a "map" of the adolescent's or adult's life experience.

Follow-up: To gain a better understanding of events that have contributed to the child's view of life and patterns of behavior.

Setting: This is a one-on-one exercise that may take up to three hours to complete.

Draw a straight line and mark off sections from birth to the current age of the child. Then ask her to tell you about any events that have been happy, sad, frightening, hurtful or made her angry during each of the years on the time line. To prevent her from becoming too overwhelmed, suggest that she only think about one year at a time, usually beginning with preschool or kindergarten. Also, if she has a hard time remembering, tell her to think about where she lived at the time, what school she went to, and who her teacher was.

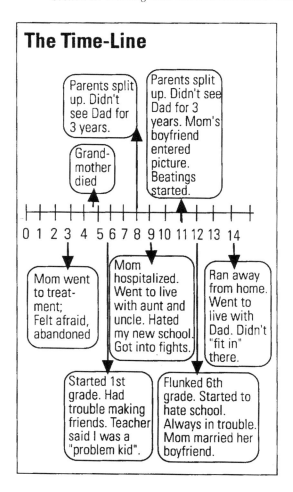

In most cases, clients have amazing recall. If they do have a hard time remembering, you may want to ask their parents to "fill in the blanks." This process can be an enlightening one for both you and your client, and it serves as a "road map" of her life that the two of you can follow that is visual and concrete.

If any of your clients report incidents of abuse (physical and/or sexual) ask them for specific details and document them in writing. If you feel the client is being truthful, then it is essential that you contact the child protective authorities in your area so that they can investigate the case and make appropriate recommendations for the child and her family.

The Thermometer

Appropriate for Ages: 6 through 9.

Materials Needed: Paper and colored pens or crayons.

Goal: To get the child to identify his level of stress compared to the stress level of other family members. (This can also be used in situations where a child is upset about a situation other than one involving his family such as a fight with a friend, conflict with several members in his class, etc.).

Follow-up: Discuss the child's level of stress and brainstorm ways he can reduce it. In cases where the child feels responsible for family problems (i.e. a divorce), acknowledge his feelings and also help him to understand that his parents are the ones who are responsible for working through the divorce.

Setting: One-on-one or in a group setting where a level of trust has been established.

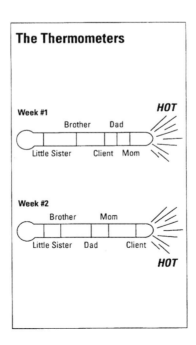

There are times when the child with FAS/FAE is unable to verbalize how upset he is. A technique that works well is the thermometer. Draw a large thermometer on a piece of paper and indicate which end means "hot." Then have the child make a mark on it that shows how "hot" he is. You may also ask him to make marks that represent how hot other family members are (using different colored pens for each family member). This gives you an idea of what the family dynamics are like and how the child with FAS/FAE feels in relation to other family members.

If there has recently been upheaval in the home, you may want to use the Thermometer drawing two weeks in a row, to see how the child is doing. His mark may be the same, even though the marks of other family members drop lower. You can then address the feelings that he continues to have, helping him work them out so that he doesn't feel so stressed.

The Body Picture

Appropriate for Ages: 4 to adult.

Materials Needed: Paper and colored pens or crayons.

Goal: To help the child identify her feelings.

Follow-up: Discuss the child's feelings with her and ways she can learn to accept and manage them.

Another technique that helps with understanding how the child with FAS/FAE feels is to draw the outline of a body (like a gingerbread man). Then have her choose four marking pens of different colors. Assign a color to four feelings: happy, angry, sad, scared. Then instruct her to fill in the body with the different colors so that you will know "how much of her" is happy, sad, angry and afraid.

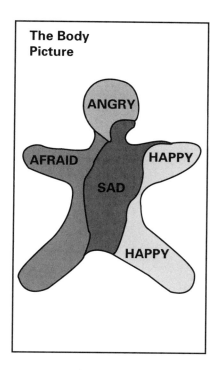

The Body Picture

ANGRY

AFRAID

HAPPY

SAD

HAPPY

Dealing with Anger

Techniques

- ❏ The Rocket Pictures
- ❏ The Volcano
- ❏ T-Shirt Exercise
- ❏ The Firecrackers
- ❏ Slugs

❑ Expressing Anger with Crayons

❑ Tearing Paper

Many children with FAS/FAE are filled with rage. So are their parents. It is so common, and yet there is a stigma attached to anger that even young children learn, early on. Children with FAS/FAE are especially prone to anger outbursts because they become frustrated so easily and they have little or no impulse control. If you begin to refer to anger as "energy" it helps to reduce the stigma. The following techniques teach children with FAS/FAE and their families how to understand their anger and deal with it in ways that won't hurt themselves or others.

The Rocket Pictures

Appropriate for Ages: 3 through 10.

Materials Needed: Paper and colored pens; or crayons; or blackboard and chalk; or wetboard and markers.

Goal: To illustrate to the child what happens when energy is directed appropriately and inappropriately.

Follow-up: To discuss instances in the child's life when they have directed their energy appropriately and inappropriately.

Setting: This can be a one-on-one or group exercise.

Draw two rockets—one going straight up, pushed by a mass of flames underneath it, and the other toppling over sideways because its flames are divided and going out to the sides. Explain to the child that the flames represent energy. When the energy goes in the direction it is supposed to (as in the picture of the first rocket) it does a good thing (like pushing the rocket straight up into the sky). However, when the energy doesn't go in the right direction, trouble occurs (like the rocket crashing).

Using the visuals of the rockets, you can begin to explore with the child how he perceives his anger. Ask him what color his anger is (most children reply that it is either

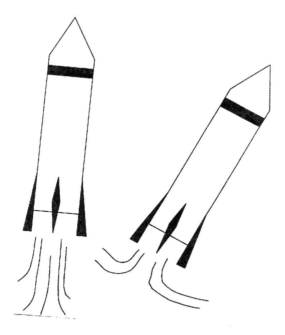

red or black) and how big it gets (it's not uncommon for a child to say his anger gets bigger than an entire room). Say that you believe that having lots of energy is good as long as it gets to come out in ways that are safe. Reassure the child that you are there to help him learn these safe ways.

For many children with FAS/FAE, having someone who talks openly about anger, and is willing to show them how to express it in positive ways is a whole new experience for them. Anger is an emotion that is just there, whether we want it to be or not. Children need adults to role model for them how to deal with their anger, and to guide them through the anger outbursts many of them often have.

The Volcano

Appropriate for Ages: 3 to adult.

Materials Needed: Paper and colored pens; or crayons; or blackboard and chalk; or wetboard and markers.

Goal: To identify what causes the child to become angry.

Follow-up: To discuss ways that anger can be worked through without an eruption having to occur.

Setting: One-on-one session or group session.

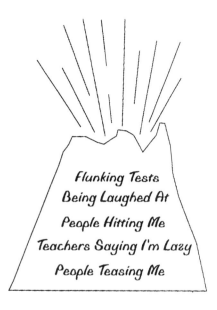

Part of learning to manage anger requires identifying what factors cause it to build up and erupt. Comparing an anger outburst to a volcano is something children can relate to. First, draw an outline of a mountain. Then ask the child what causes a mountain to become a volcano. (Most children say that pressure builds up inside the mountain and then the pressure blows the top off it.)

You can then say that the same thing happens when people get mad. Things build up inside of them and they explode. With some people, it doesn't take much to make them blow up. With others, it takes more things and a longer time.

At this point, draw several straight lines inside the outline of the mountain. Ask the child to tell you some of the things that make her angry and write them down on the lines. Say that the things you have listed for her are just like the pressures that build up inside a volcanic mountain. Commend the child for helping you better understand her anger and encourage her to keep the picture and continue adding to the list so that she becomes more aware of what triggers her off and why. Each time you work with her, the two of you can go over the list, decide on ways that the pressure can be released before it gets to the point of explosion, and what to do if the child does explode.

It is important, too, that other adults who are regularly in contact with the child be informed of strategies you and she have discussed. They can then remind the child of these strategies whenever it looks as though she is about to lose her temper and explode. Sometimes just saying "Remember the volcano," snaps the child out of it long enough for her to collect herself and choose a more appropriate way to express anger.

T-Shirt Exercise

Appropriate for Ages: 8-Adolescent.

Materials Needed: Light, solid-colored T-shirt, laundry marker, or butcher paper cut into size of a T-shirt and marking pens.

Goal: For child to identify her likes and dislikes and then communicate these facts by writing them out on her T-shirt.

Follow-up: Discuss the likes and dislikes of the child.

Setting: One-on-one or group.

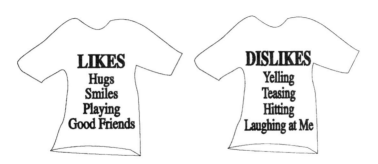

LIKES
Hugs
Smiles
Playing
Good Friends

DISLIKES
Yelling
Teasing
Hitting
Laughing at Me

Tell the child to pretend that she is going to a party where she has to let others know what she likes and dislikes, but she cannot speak to them. Instead, she will write what she likes and dislikes on the front and back of her shirt. One side is for the "likes" and the other side is for the "dislikes." Other topics that can be used include: Strengths vs. Improvements in Progress; Ways You'll Know I'm Happy and Ways You'll Know I'm Sad; and Goals I've Achieved vs. Goals I Want To Achieve.

Another way to do this exercise in a group setting is to have the participants write descriptions of themselves on the front and back of slips of paper. Then have them put the slips of paper into a basket or bag and have one designated person draw the slips out, one at a time, and read them aloud. The rest of the group then tries to guess which description was written by whom.

The Firecrackers

Appropriate for Ages: 6 through 12.

Materials Needed: Paper and colored pens or crayons; or blackboard and chalk; or wetboard and markers.

Goal: To illustrate how people, just like firecrackers, can either have a short temper (short fuse) or are slow to anger (long fuse).

Follow-up: To discuss the type of fuse the child has, why he may have that type of fuse, and the consequences or outcome of his having it. If the child is short-tempered, ways can be discussed to help him with better impulse control and appropriate outlets for releasing his energy. If the child has a long fuse, the difference between healthy impulse control and "stuffing" anger should be discussed.

Setting: One-on-one or group exercise.

A child with FAS/FAE who has a tendency toward anger outbursts needs to find ways to "lengthen his fuse." Have him draw two firecrackers—one with a long fuse and one with a short one. Then begin a discussion about how

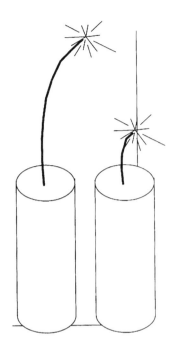

some firecrackers take longer to explode than others. Explain that people can be much like firecrackers in that some of them get angry very quickly and others don't. Ask him which firecracker he would be. Then ask him why he thinks that. Encourage him to write down the things (or situations) that cause him to "explode" quickly, and what he can do to "lengthen his fuse."

I once observed a boy who was considered to have a "short fuse" patiently working on a model car. He took great care in putting the car together and didn't seem to get frustrated even when, at first, some of the car parts were difficult to put together.

After he finished his project, I commented on how patient he had been. I said, "I noticed that when you were working on the model you were very patient. I admire that! It seems to me that if you are able to have a long fuse in this area of your life, then that means we can work on transferring some of that patience over into other areas of your life, too. For instance, I bet you can use your 'long fuse ability' to manage your anger better."

He had never made that connection before, but thought it was an idea worth trying.

Slugs

Appropriate for Ages: 3 to adult.

Materials Needed: Paper and colored pens or crayons; or large sheet of tag board; or 2 sheets of colored paper, scissors, paste, marking pens or crayons (the outline of a slug can be cut out of tag board or a smaller version of a slug out of one piece of colored paper and pasted on to the second piece of colored paper).

Goal: To enable clients to identify what things "hurt their feelings" (inside hurts).

Follow-up: To discuss the inside hurts they have identified and to encourage them to:

1. Acknowledge their inside hurts,
2. Decide who they can go to talk about their inside hurts,
3. Learn to verbalize their inside hurts to the people they trust and who can help them to process these hurts.

Setting: One-on-one or group exercise.

Very often the emotion that causes anger is hurt. There are two kinds of hurt—"inside hurts" and "outside hurts." Outside hurts are things like bumps, bruises, scrapes, scratches, lumps, and other marks that let people know that a person has been hurt. Inside hurts, however, are connected with how that person may feel or react inside to something that is said or done to them.

An example I have used to represent inside hurts is a rubber slug. (For those of you who live in regions where there aren't any slugs, they are slimy, crawling mollusks that are common in the Northwest.) Slugs are sticky and inside hurts also have a tendency to "stick" to a person.

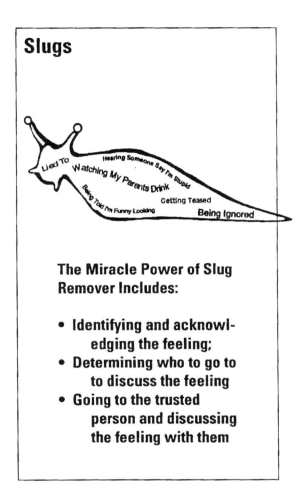

Slugs

Lied To

Hearing Someone Say I'm Stupid

Watching My Parents Drink

Being Told I'm Funny Looking

Getting Teased

Being Ignored

The Miracle Power of Slug Remover Includes:

- **Identifying and acknowledging the feeling;**
- **Determining who to go to to discuss the feeling**
- **Going to the trusted person and discussing the feeling with them**

You might want to describe to the child what some common inside hurts are: being made fun of, feeling left out, getting a poor grade on a test, etc. Then ask the child what some of her inside hurts are. You may even want to have her draw a large slug and list her inside hurts inside the slug (much like the volcano technique). Again, she can add more inside hurts to the list as she becomes aware of them.

As you talk to the child about her inside hurts, let her know that she possesses "the miracle power of slug remover." In fact, tell her that she has just used her power by talking to you about what hurts her feelings. Removing slugs requires talking about her inside hurts rather than stuffing them inside herself so that they build up and eventually cause an anger outburst (or illness and/or depression).

Together, the two of you can discuss the different people that she knows she can talk to and who she can count on for understanding and support. Children with FAS/FAE often get their feelings hurt. Slugs are creatures they can remember and who help them learn to talk about the inside hurts they are experiencing. If you are working with a group of children on a regular basis, you can establish a ritual of having "slug removal time" at the beginning of your group sessions. One group leader had her students make large cardboard slugs with lists of various kinds of inside hurts. Each time her group met, she passed the slugs out to the children and then walked around the group with a gallon-sized plastic bag and instructed the children to verbalize what their most recent inside hurts were, as they put their slugs into the bag. By doing this exercise, she was giving them permission to acknowledge their "inside hurts," providing them with the opportunity to talk through their feelings, and helping them learn coping skills should the inside hurts happen again.

Expressing Anger with Crayons

Appropriate for Ages: 3 through 10.

Materials Needed: Butcher paper to cover a tabletop, masking tape, extra large crayons.

Goal: To express anger in a positive way.

Setting: One-on-one.

Follow-up: Discuss what is causing the anger.

Cover a table or a large portion of a table with butcher paper. Tape the paper to the table. Encourage the child to

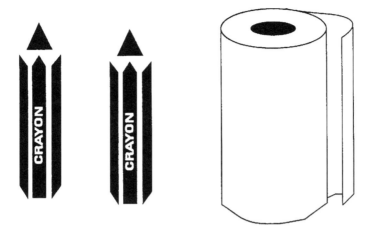

choose a large crayon for each hand, then tell him he is free to scribble all over the paper, as a way for him to get his anger out. As he does so, act as his "cheering section" by saying things like: "Go ahead, get it out," "Good job—you're getting a lot of mean feelings out," etc.

Tearing Paper

Appropriate for All Ages

Materials Needed: Newspaper or paper later used for paper mache projects.

Goal: To release anger.

Follow-up: To discuss the cause of the anger.

Setting: A space where others won't be disturbed by the noise.

Give the child a large amount of paper and let her tear it up. Let her know that this is an appropriate way to release her energy/anger. Compliment her on her ability to do so.

Ways of Releasing Energy

Techniques

❏ Bats and Balloons

❏ Hanging Balloons

❏ Blowing Up a Balloon

❏ Balloons on a Rubber Band

❏ The Crib Mattress

❏ The Mini-Trampoline

❏ The Rocket Room

The list of physical ways to release energy can go on and on. In addition to the techniques in this book, you could try—

Pounding on pillows

Shooting baskets

Doing push-ups

Lifting weights

Hitting a tether ball

Swimming

Running laps

Jumping rope

Chopping wood (always with supervision)

Find out from the children you live and work with what works best for them. Many children with FAS/FAE are hyperactive to begin with, plus they are constantly having to deal with frustrations and disappointments. Allowing them to release their anger and energy is so important. Balloons, bats, boxing gloves, a crib mattress or big pillows, a mini-trampoline and other physical activities give them permission and provide them with opportunities to do this.

To help reduce agitation, some parents and teachers have provided their children with bubble packaging material and large aquarium tubing. Children like to pop the packaging bubbles and chew on the aquarium tubing when they feel like shouting or biting.

Bats and Balloons

Appropriate for Ages: 2 to adult.

Materials Needed: two plastic baseball bats, one balloon.

Goal: To release energy.

Follow-up: To discuss how energy can be released in a positive way; to identify who the child may be mad at or what they are upset about in order to problem-solve the situation.

Setting: A large space for the one-on-one exchange.

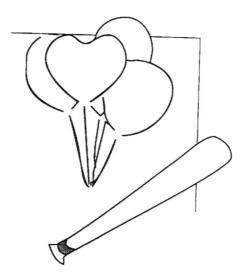

Using two plastic baseball bats and a large balloon is a wonderful way to put a child at ease, get him to talk to you, and help him release his anger. This technique is especially effective when meeting with a child for the first time or getting two children to work out a conflict.

Tell the child you'd like to take a few minutes to just play. Hand him a bat and then hit the balloon to him with your bat. It's difficult for anyone to miss a balloon so when he hits it back, comment on his powerful swing, good form, etc. After the two of you have volleyed the balloon back and forth a few times, you might mention that when you are angry or feeling a lot of energy about something, hitting the balloon is one of the ways you get your anger/energy out. Then ask the child if he ever feels angry about something. Suggest that he pretend that the balloon represents something or someone he gets mad at. Then encourage him to hit the balloon as hard as he can until he feels that he has gotten much of his energy out.

If you are working with a child in a school setting and he is having a conflict with another student, talk to both children separately and then let them hit the balloon back and forth to each other. Usually it greatly diffuses their anger and gives you an opportunity to help them problem-solve their dispute.

Children respond well to the bats and balloons technique, not only because it is fun and puts them at ease with you, but also because it allows them to work through their anger in a non-destructive way. They know they can come to you and admit they are angry, and you will not judge them or try to get them to repress it. The more they get to know you, the more they will tell you about their other feelings, as well.

Hanging Balloons

Appropriate for Ages: 2 through 10.

Materials Needed: Balloons and string (and something to hang them from).

Goal: To release energy.

Follow-up: To discuss what the energy is about—anger, frustration, etc.

Setting: A large space.

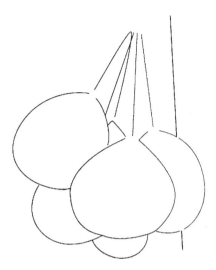

With a younger child, blow up a half dozen balloons, tie them together, and hang them upside down from the ceiling. Then let the child hit the bunch of balloons with the bat. The goal here is to let the child get her energy out before you try to talk with her about what is making her angry.

Blowing Up a Balloon

Appropriate for Ages: 6 to adult.

Materials Needed: One balloon.

Goal: To release energy.

Follow-up: To discuss what the energy is about.

Setting: One-on-one (with supervision if the child is under 12).

A third grader once told me that when he got angry he would blow into a large balloon, pretending that each puff was helping to release his anger. "I blow my anger into the balloon until the balloon gets full," he said. "Then if I still feel angry, I let all the air out of the balloon and start over again."

Balloon on a Rubber Band

Appropriate for Ages: 2 to adult.

Materials Needed: One large, heavy-duty balloon with long rubber band.

Goal: To release energy.

Follow-up: To discuss what the energy is about.

Setting: One-on-one.

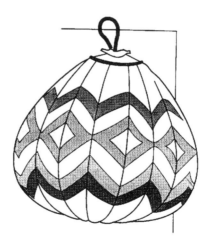

This type of balloon is excellent for using with two plastic bats. There are also larger, "heavy duty" balloons that come with long, thick rubber bands that can be attached to the balloons. When the balloons are blown up, children can then punch them repeatedly. These balloons also work well with plastic bats. Because they are almost the size of beach balls, they are easy to hit, and they last a long time.

Whenever children play with balloons, there should be supervision, especially if the children are blowing the balloons up. There is always the risk that the balloon may be swallowed or the rubber used for snapping another person.

The Crib Mattress

Appropriate for Ages: 3 through 12.

Materials Needed: Crib mattress, boxing gloves, plastic bat, blanket (if mattress is used for comforting).

Goal: To release energy.

Follow-up: To discuss the cause of their anger and ways they can get it out without hitting others and/or hurting themselves or destroying property.

Setting: A private room or area for this one-on-one activity.

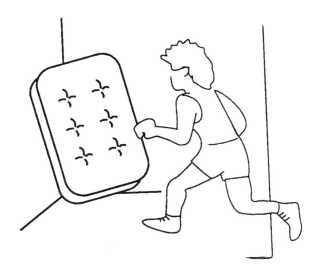

A crib mattress serves as an inexpensive substitute for a punching bag. Often you can find one in a second-hand shop. It's best if it has a plain, plastic cover so children can draw and write on it with magic markers. (My students drew the outline of a person on both sides of the mattress. Then they identified the places on the body where children usually get hurt or abused. Also, when they were mad at a particular person they would write his or her name on the mattress, giving me more insight into whom they got angry at the most.)

Provide one set of boxing gloves for the child to use on the mattress, if she wishes. Some children prefer to punch the mattress with their bare fists, kick it, throw it around, or hit it with the plastic bat.

Let them know that the mattress is there for them to let their energy out on, and when they have done so, then you are there to listen to them explain how they are feeling and why. Children often need to physically "vent" before they can verbalize what is making them angry. When they are in a calmer state (and it doesn't take long for them to de-escalate with the crib mattress), they are more open to hearing what you have to say. (Some children may want to use the mattress to lie down or curl up on. Have a blanket handy for instances like this.)

The Mini-Trampoline

Appropriate for Ages: 2-1/2 to adult.

Materials Needed: Mini-trampoline.

Goal: To release energy.

Follow-up: To discuss what the energy is about.

Setting: Use a private room or area for this one-on-one activity. Always supervise children under 12.

Mini-trampolines also help children release energy. One of the mothers of an FAE child found that when her son began to escalate, it helped if she had him jump on the family's mini-trampoline. She took the time to supervise him when he did this. After he was through jumping, she talked things over with him.

The Rocket Room

Appropriate for Ages: 2 to adult.

Materials Needed: Bats and balloons, pillows, punching bag, boxing gloves, mini-trampoline, etc.

Goal: To have a safe place to go for releasing energy in appropriate ways.

Follow-up: To discuss what the energy is about.

Setting: A specific room in the home, school or treatment facility where supervision is provided when necessary (especially with children ages 2 through 10).

Having a room set up in your home or school where children with FAS/FAE can go specifically to release their energy is ideal. One family I worked with turned a room in their house into what they called "The Rocket Room." They had a mini-trampoline in there, as well as large pillows and two plastic bats and a beach ball. Originally it was set up for their four-year-old FAE son, but soon all family members used it, including Mom and Dad when they were feeling angry. The parents reported that having the Rocket Room really made a difference in how the whole family began to relate. The parents felt that they were being positive role models for all of their children because they were learning to release more of their own tension, and as a result, were also able to relate better to each other.

A Squeeze Toy

Appropriate for All Ages.

Materials Needed: 6 inch balloon, funnel, measuring cup, spoon, flour.

Goal: To make a squeeze toy to be used for release of energy/agitation.

Follow-up: Discuss situations when this toy will come in handy. Stress that it is a good prevention against anger outbursts.

Setting: One-on-one or group.

Measure approximately 1/3 cup of flour. Insert funnel into the neck of the balloon. Slowly spoon the flour into the balloon, filling its round space completely. Tie knot in the neck of the balloon. It is now ready to be squeezed in times of stress.

Techniques for Building Self-Esteem

Techniques

❑ Computer and the Printer

❑ The Little Green Guy

❑ The Boom Box

❑ The On/Off Switch

❑ Personal Books

❑ The Bare Wire

❑ What's the Beef?

❑ The Thinking Cap

Computer and the Printer

When a phrase is programmed into a computer over and over again, what message will the printer print out? Too often, we adults think that if we constantly remind a child of his shortcomings, this will somehow inspire him to change and become more like the person we want him to become. Not so. The messages we input into a child are usu-

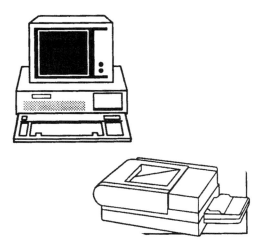

ally what they act out. Children with FAS/FAE go through their lives hearing almost daily how they aren't measuring up. This erodes their self-esteem and they become very discouraged. They need to hear more about what they are doing well and given opportunities to succeed both at home and at school.

The Little Green Guy

Appropriate for Ages: 3 to adult.

Materials Needed: An ugly finger puppet that is green.

Goal: To teach the concept of negative self-talk by using a visual image that children, adolescents and adults can relate to.

Follow-up: To identify and discuss negative messages and replace them with positive messages.

Setting: One-on-one or group sessions.

Children with FAS/FAE often have poor judgment. Left unsupervised, they can get into trouble. It may not be until "after the fact" that they realize that they have done some-

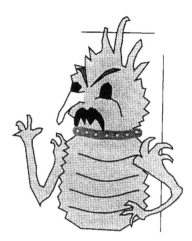

thing wrong. Sometimes they don't even understand what "wrong" is.

For those children who do have some concept of wrong, the Little Green Guy helps them to think more about their actions. He is a finger puppet with big eyes and an angry expression on his face. He can be compared to Oscar the Grouch on the Sesame Street television show.

You may choose a finger puppet of another color and design but the message you want to get across is that the Little Green Guy likes to encourage the child to get into trouble. He always has a good argument as to why the child should do the wrong thing and he is very convincing. However, whenever the child gets caught, the Little Green Guy just laughs and ridicules him.

"Ha, ha, ha, there you go again. You got caught, didn't you? You are so stupid. Ha, ha, ha."

The Little Green Guy is an unhappy, angry character and he likes to see other people feeling the same way. Being just a finger puppet, though, he doesn't have to be allowed as much power as he would like to have. You can say to the child with FAS/FAE you are working with, "Who is bigger, you or this finger puppet? He has no right to boss you around or say things to put you down. You are the boss of him. When you start thinking about doing something wrong, think about The Little Green Guy and how you are in charge. And when other people say or do mean things to you, remember that they have Little Green Guys, too, and they haven't learned how to be in charge of their Little Green Guys, yet." Help the child with FAS/FAE to associate doing something wrong with a character (visual and concrete) that they can remember.

The Boom Box

Appropriate for Ages: 9 through 12.

Materials Needed: Paper, colored pens, crayons.

Goal: To help clients identify the negative messages that they are used to hearing and how they can turn them into more positive messages.

Follow-up: discussion of negative and positive messages and the feelings the child associates with them.

Setting: One-on-one or group activity.

The Boom Box

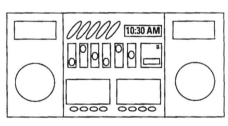

Green Guy Tape

You Are Stupid
You Can't Do Any-
thing
Nobody Loves You
You Are A Trouble-
maker

Positive Tape

I Am Smart in Lots
of Ways
I Can Do Many
Things Well
My Mom and Dad
Love Me
I am Good at Using
My Off Switch

Music is in the lives of most children with FAS/FAE. They know when a tape in a cassette player (or boom box) doesn't sound right and they know when to replace it with one that does. This exercise is a good one to use after talking to a child about his Little Green Guy. Have him draw a boom box for you. Then instruct him to draw pictures of two cassette tapes—one on one side of the boom box and one on the other. Next, have him identify several things that his Little Green Guy might say to him to make him feel bad about himself or to cause him to get into trouble. Have him list those things under one of the cassette tape drawings. Then, taking one phrase at a time, ask him what he would rather hear and have him list these things under the second cassette.

Tell him that the first cassette could be called "The Little Green Guy Tape"—one that he certainly wouldn't want to have to listen to over and over again. Point out to him that he has the power to "stop that tape" and replace it with the second one which is much more positive and makes him feel better about himself.

It is good to inform parents and teachers about this technique because often children with FAS/FAE get many of their Little Green Guy messages from home and school. Positive self-talk builds healthy self-esteem. Children with FAS/FAE need others to constantly remind them that they have strengths and are lovable. They need to have strong self-esteem messages repeated to them often, because they aren't always capable of remembering how to do their own positive self-talk. This exercise can be done as a large poster to be hung in a place where it is frequently seen and can serve as a reminder that Little Green Guy tapes can be replaced by ones that sound much better.

The Off/On Switch

Appropriate for Ages: 5 through 12.

Materials Needed: An electric off/on switch.

Goal: To illustrate impulse control.

Follow-up: Identify actions that reflect no impulse control and actions that do. To then discuss ways in which impulses can be more successfully controlled.

Setting: One-on-one or group sessions.

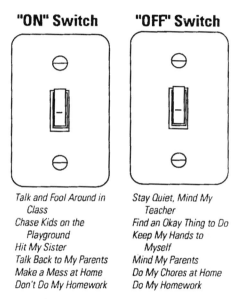

"ON" Switch	"OFF" Switch
Talk and Fool Around in Class	Stay Quiet, Mind My Teacher
Chase Kids on the Playground	Find an Okay Thing to Do
Hit My Sister	Keep My Hands to Myself
Talk Back to My Parents	Mind My Parents
Make a Mess at Home	Do My Chores at Home
Don't Do My Homework	Do My Homework

Lack of impulse control is another characteristic of children with FAS/FAE. The Off/On switch technique can be used when a behavior is beginning to escalate and intervention is necessary. During a time when your child with FAS/FAE is in a calm, receptive mood, show her an electrical light switch and say, "Do you know that you have a switch, just like this one, inside of you? Yes, you do! It is invisible but it really works—especially when you are reminded that you are about to do something you shouldn't be doing and then you decide not to. When you stop doing the wrong thing, it's like flipping your switch off. If you go ahead and do the wrong thing, then that means you left the switch on."

Have a light switch available so that the child can actually hold it in her hand as you teach her this technique. (The uninstalled switch seems to have more impact than one that is already in the wall because it is unusual to look at.) Also, have the child draw a switch that is on and then a second switch that is off. Under the "On" switch have her list some of the things that commonly get her into trouble, and under the "off" switch, have her list the things she does to stop herself from getting into trouble.

The off/on switch is extremely popular with children. They like to tell other children about it, and it is not uncommon for them to say, "My off switch isn't working very well today, so I've come to you to ask for help so that it will be fixed and I won't get into trouble."

If you see a child's behavior escalating, you can say, "Use your off switch!" and they often respond by stopping what they are doing. A group of children may remind each other to use their off switches. Several boys in a second grade class actually formed a "club" to spread the word about the off switch around school and to keep each other out of trouble.

Personal Books

Appropriate for Ages: 3 to adult.

Materials Needed: Tag board, colored and/or ruled paper, colored pens, string or staples for binding the book, a personal photograph or pictures cut from magazines.

Goal: To build self-esteem in the child and to help the adult working with the child on this project to gain insights into the child's thoughts, feelings, strengths and weaknesses. Also, to serve as a catalyst for discussion between the child and the adult.

Follow-up: To discuss the contents of each page.

Setting: One-on-one is preferable, but it can be done as a group project where everyone gets individual time with an adult.

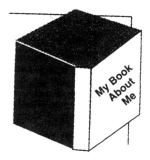

Making a personal book for a child with FAS/FAE is another way to build his self-esteem. Together you and the child can decide what to include in the book, such as his strengths, ways he takes good care of himself, names of people he loves and who love him, how he can stay safe, who he can go to for help, etc.

One child was so proud of his completed book that he asked me when I was going to take a picture of him.

"What do you mean?" I asked.

"Well," he replied, "all authors have their pictures on the back of their books."

A personal book makes a child with FAS/FAE feel special. Depending on what the child writes, the book can serve as a "guidebook" and source of comfort when he feels bad and needs reassurance. It can also be an ongoing project with new pages added on a regular basis. The experience of putting such a book together can be a very empowering one for a child with FAS/FAE.

The Bare Wire *(for the Child Who Feels Like a Victim)*

Appropriate for Ages: 8 to adult.

Materials Needed: A wire with insulation.

Goal: To illustrate what it looks like to be unprotected.

Follow-up: To talk about how and why the child feels like a victim and to brainstorm ways that she can insulate herself.

Setting: One-on-one.

Children with FAS/FAE often feel like victims. They are teased, laughed at, rejected and taken advantage of. Those with higher IQs know that they are different and feel helpless to do anything about it. The bare wire technique acknowledges how they must feel and reassures them that there are ways they can protect themselves.

Take a piece of insulated wire and strip the protective covering off one end of it so that the bare wire is exposed. Show this wire to the child with FAS/FAE and say, "I can imagine that you must feel like this part of the wire that has no covering—no insulation on it. That can't be a very good feeling at all. I would like to help you find ways to protect yourself, just like the insulation protects this wire."

As you get to know the child better, you can find out what makes her feel unsafe and what she has been doing to protect herself so far. Also find out who she feels good around (who is caring and supportive) and what kind of supervision she gets. Let her know that you want to help her build a network of people whose caring can offset the words and actions of those who are insensitive, and that you also want to help her find additional ways to comfort herself.

Talking with parents and teachers of the child can give you a clearer picture of what kinds of stresses the child is facing every day. Include them in the "insulation building" process so that the child feels she has additional support. Discuss, too, the possibility of closer supervision so that she isn't further victimized, which often happens as the child gets older and more is expected of her.

Conflict Resolution—What's the Beef?

Appropriate for Ages: 6 to adult.

Materials Needed: A plastic hamburger that can be taken apart (or one made out of cardboard or other art supplies).

Goal: To illustrate what a conflict "looks" like.

Follow-up: To discuss how a specific conflict can be resolved.

Setting: Effective to use when a conflict arises between two people.

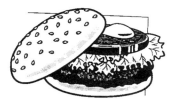

Conflict can come up frequently in the lives of children with FAS/FAE. When this occurs, showing them how to focus on the main issue, rather than all the details and who is to blame, can be beneficial.

To help you illustrate your point, use a plastic hamburger that comes apart. Pick up the beef and say, "What's the beef—the main thing you and the other person(s) are having a conflict about?" Then, pick up the bun and say, "The top half of this bun is you and the bottom half is the other person. The two of you are caught up in a beef." (Then put the beef between the buns.) "The tomato, lettuce, pickles, cheese, etc. are all the details that the two of you are giving me, including who you feel is to blame. But you know what? I'm not interested in all the details and who is to blame. I'm interested in hearing how you think you can settle this conflict and not have it happen again. Let's look closely at the beef and figure out how to solve the problem it has caused."

The Thinking Cap

Appropriate for Ages: 6 through 10.

Materials Needed: A very unique kind of hat or cap.

Goal: To motivate the child to think carefully about what you have asked him and to show that you believe he has the answer to your question.

Follow-up: To discuss his answer(s).

Setting: One-on-one.

A common response from children who are asked to answer questions, including how to solve their problems, is "I don't know." To counter this, you may say, "I believe you do. In fact, I think kids are very smart and have lots of good answers. Here, let's put the thinking cap on your head and give it a few minutes to work. It will stir the information up in your brain and then I bet you'll know."

A "thinking cap" can be any kind of clever-looking cap that children perceive as magical. The one I use is a visor cap that has lights that blink on it when it is hooked up to a battery attached to the headband. Young children love it and invariably come up with an answer within one to two minutes. Older children say, "okay, okay, I'll tell you. I don't want to wear that thing!"

What the children respond to mostly, is the strong message that they *do* have the answers and that their answers *matter.* Even if a child with FAS/FAE is especially intellectually impaired, I still like to give him a positive message about knowing the answers. This seems far more appropriate to me than saying something like, "Well, I realize you are not very bright, so there is no point in expecting you to problem-solve."

Behavior Modification Techniques

Techniques:

❏ The Listening Room/Special Corner/Office Space

❏ Sticker Charts

❏ The Clipboard

❏ Hand Drawing

❏ Using a Sleeping Bag, Blanket, or Weighted Apron

❏ The Hour Glass

The Angry, Disruptive Child in the Classroom

As has been mentioned earlier, it is not uncommon for students with FAS/FAE to have anger outbursts. They can become easily frustrated and that, coupled with their low impulse control, can quickly "set them off." When an outburst occurs, certain strategies need to be used:

❏ Remove the child from anyone else who may be around (or ask the others to leave)

❏ Allow the child to "cool down" before trying to talk to her. If the child tends to be very physical, suggest that she release some energy in an appropriate way (e.g., by throwing a ball against a wall, running around the track, hitting a tether ball, shooting baskets, jumping rope, pounding on a pillow). The child should be supervised during this period of time

❏ Do not attempt to physically subdue the child unless it is absolutely necessary. Instead, tell her that you know she can get herself under control

❏ When speaking to her, do so in a soft, steady tone of voice. Do not attempt to berate her or lecture her. This will only escalate her anger

❏ When she calms down, discuss with her what she has done. "Walk her through" the details that led up to the episode. Ask her how she could have done things differently. Then ask her how she is prepared to handle a similar situation, should it happen in the future

❏ If there is a consequence for the inappropriate behavior, carry it out

If the event involves another student, wait until they both cool down and then bring them together to discuss what happened and how they can do things differently if it should happen again. Keep in mind that it will be necessary to continue to repeat to the student with FAS/FAE ways that she can better handle her anger. Going over it only once will not ensure that the child has "gotten it."

When dealing with a student who is usually quiet and withdrawn, but who periodically has an anger outburst, the same guidelines can be followed. This particular kind of student may want to calm himself down in a quieter way, but one never knows for sure. Whenever an outburst does occur, it is best to follow your instinct regarding how to handle the situation. A student may want to physically release anger one day and be alone to calm down the next. Having a place where either method can be used is highly recommended. Some ways of encouraging children to calm down include:

❑ Deep breathing

❑ Listening to soft music

❑ Drawing

❑ Rocking

❑ Looking at books

Again, it is important that the child has someone to talk to, once he gets himself under control, preferably someone he knows and trusts.

Discipline Versus Punishment

Children with FAS/FAE need to be held responsible for their actions, even if they have difficulty distinguishing right from wrong. However, there is a difference between discipline and punishment. Discipline involves a natural consequence that is related to the inappropriate behavior of the child. Punishment, on the other hand, implies that the child is "bad," and guilt and shame are used to attempt to change the child's behavior.

Punishment may alter a child's behavior for the moment, but it also breeds resentment, hatred, and rage. She will spend time thinking up ways to "get back" at the person who has punished her, rather than thinking about what she has done wrong.

Many times inappropriate behavior from a child with FAS/FAE can be avoided by providing constant supervision and not setting up situations where she is likely to get into trouble. When there are incidents, discipline should be fair. You may also want to ask yourself:

❑ Could this incident have been avoided with more adult supervision?

❑ Are my expectations too high for this child?

❑ Is this something that has happened before and am I expecting the child to react in a different way because we talked about it then? (In other words, am I expecting this child to remember something when she may not be able to retain things for very long?)

Depending on the level of intelligence and the emotional development of the child, sometimes we can include them in the process of determining consequences. Often this is done during a time when the child is calm and receptive. Let her decide what the consequences should be for which behaviors. Make a chart that has the actions and the consequences listed on it. Then, if an incident does occur, you can simply refer to the chart and say, "According to what you decided, the consequence for this is such-and-such."

Putting the responsibility of the consequence back onto the child avoids your being blamed or resented for coming up with one that she might feel is unfair. You may still have to make sure that the consequence is enforced, but at least the child has had a role in the process.

It is also important that there be a "united front" when more than one adult is involved in the disciplining of a child. Whether it be two or more staff members or two parents (or primary caretakers), they should support one another in being clear and fair with the child. It is also essential that they be consistent. If a child senses that one adult is strict and the other is permissive, then much manipulation, on the child's part, is likely to occur. When there is not a united front, children are more likely to continue their inappropriate behaviors.

The Listening Room/Special Corner/Office Space

Giving children a time-out has become a popular way of disciplining. However, many children with FAS/FAE feel a degree of shame when they are told to take a time-out because they see themselves as "bad." Providing an area where they can go to calm down and collect themselves is a positive alternative to a time-out. Let them know that the room or corner is a special place where they can "listen to themselves." You might say, "Sometimes we just need to get away from everyone and be very quiet. Then we can figure out what's the matter and what will make things better."

One teacher converted a closet in her room into a "Listening Room" where students could go, sit quietly, and think about what was upsetting them. The room had a chair in it and the walls were painted blue with clouds and rainbows.

Another teacher created an "Office Space" for her student with FAS. She provided him with a desk that he could work at when he needed to be separate from the rest of the class. A file cabinet blocked his view of the classroom. This arrangement helped him to focus better.

A Special Corner might have items such as a pillow, blanket, books, a teddy bear, a Walkman that plays soothing music, a rocking chair, etc. More active toys (plastic bats, crib mattress, boxing gloves, etc.) should be in the counselor's office or someplace else away from the classroom. (As was mentioned earlier, an extremely angry child needs to be supervised away from his classmates while he releases his energy.)

Whatever type of area or room you decide upon, don't make it a punitive place. Students who go there need to feel that it is a privilege to do so and to know that once they calm down, an adult will take the time to talk things through with them.

Sticker Charts

Appropriate for Ages: 3 to adult.

Materials Needed: Large piece of paper or tagboard, colorful stickers.

Goal: To encourage the child/adolescent/adult to earn stickers for good behavior.

Follow-up: Acknowledge the good behavior after each sticker is attained and follow through with a prize of some kind, once a certain number of stickers have been earned.

Setting: One-on-one interaction.

Children with FAS/FAE respond especially well to sticker charts. They like to know what is expected of them and be able to actually see the results of their improved behavior. It is important that you include these children in the individual planning of what goes on their charts (the behaviors they want to change and what they need from others to help them do so.) Also, it helps if you don't have too many goals listed on the charts at once and that stickers are given daily, rather than making children wait too long to be rewarded. You may even want to break the day into hours or half-days and make check marks that count towards earning stickers. (See also sample on page 110.)

Rewards for earning stickers can range from certain privileges (watching T.V., going out for a meal, renting a video) to buying children toys. This technique is most effective when parents and teachers work together to reinforce positive behaviors. Children with FAS/FAE need to know that the expectations for them are consistent both at school and at home.

The Clipboard

Appropriate for Ages: 8 to adult.

Materials Needed: Clipboard, paper, pen or pencil (attached to the clipboard).

	Homework In	Listened Well	Hands To Self	Good Bus Behavior
Mon.			Hit Shannon	
Tue.			Pushed Montez	Got Out Of Seat During Ride
Wed.		Talked To Jason When It Was Teacher's Turn		
Thur.				
Fri.		Made Noises When You Should Have Been Listening	Took Pencil From Paul's Desk	

Goal: To encourage appropriate behavior and/or completed assignments.

Follow-up: Praise the child/adolescent/adult whenever a goal on the chart has been met.

Setting: One-on-one interaction.

Another way to measure progress, raise self-esteem, and monitor behaviors of children with FAS/FAE at school is to use the clipboard technique. The clipboard is much like a sticker chart only it is carried around by the child with FAS/FAE at school and teachers "sign off" when the student meets the criteria listed on the clipboard sheet. The student with FAS/FAE likes the attention she gets when her clipboard paper is signed. She can look at it frequently to stay on track and to see proof of her progress.

Hand Drawing

Appropriate for Ages: 5 through 8.

Materials Needed: Paper, marking pens.

Goal: To help child realize that hands are not for hurting others.

Follow-up: To discuss positive reasons for using hands and to discourage using hands for hurting.

Setting: One-on-one or group.

Have the child put one of her hands on a piece of paper and trace its outline. Then have her do the same thing with the other hand. Tell her how nice you think her hands are and ask her why she thinks people have hands—what are some ways that hands are used? Write her answers down on the same piece of paper. Hopefully, most of her answers will be positive ones such as: "To eat with," "To throw a ball," "To turn pages," etc. Focus on the answers that are positive and say: "I am glad to hear what you think hands are for, instead of for hitting, pinching, slapping, etc. Doing mean things

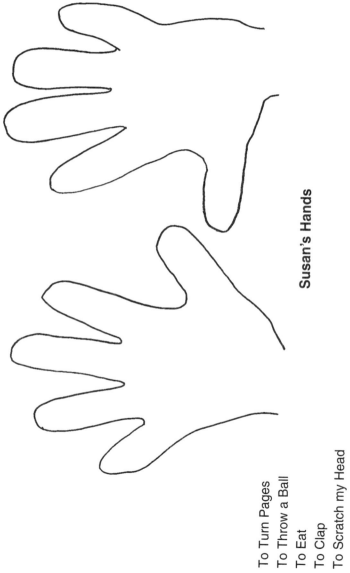

Susan's Hands

To Turn Pages
To Throw a Ball
To Eat
To Clap
To Scratch my Head

with your hands will hurt others and probably get you into trouble. It's good for you to remember all the nice and useful things that you think hands are for. I am proud of the things you have thought of that are good, nice and useful."

Encourage the child to keep her hand drawing in a place where she can look at it often so she can remember what the two of you have talked about. Suggest to her that looking at her drawing regularly will help her to do nice and useful things with her hands, rather than hurtful things.

Using a Sleeping Bag, Blanket, or Weighted Apron

Appropriate for Ages: 2 to adolescent.

Materials Needed: Sleeping bag, blanket, or weighted apron.

Goal: To calm the child.

Follow-up: Dialogue with the child, once he has calmed down.

Setting: A quiet space in the room for the individual child.

Teachers and parents have reported that often children are able to calm themselves if they can feel physically safe by wrapping themselves up in a sleeping bag or blanket, or by putting on an apron that has been weighted down. In one therapeutic preschool setting, the teacher had an old lead dental apron that was used when patients had x-rays taken of their teeth. She discovered that the children would ask if they could put the apron on whenever they felt agitated and needed to get themselves under control. The weight of the apron was a comfort to them in that it enabled them to sit or lie still.

Likewise, sleeping bags and blankets help children feel safe and more in control of their physical well-being (as if they were in a cocoon) when they wrap themselves up in them. Or, an apron can be made with pockets of sand sewn into it in strategic places.

Hour Glass

Appropriate for Ages: 3 through 10.

Materials Needed: Two plastic liter bottles, narrow funnel, sand, strong tape.

Goal: To use in situations where the child needs to become focused and calm.

Follow-up: Check to see how the child is doing. Acknowledge her ability to calm herself down by focusing on the bottles of sand.

Setting: A quiet space in the room for the individual child.

Fill one liter bottle almost to the top with sand. Fit a narrow funnel into its mouth, and then tape the two bottle mouths together. (The funnel should be very narrow so that sand passes through it slowly.) Invert the bottles so that the sand will run down into the second bottle. The narrower the funnel, the longer it will take for the sand to fill the second bottle, thus giving the child adequate time to calm down. The child may need to reverse the bottles and do deep breathing exercises a number of times before she is ready to rejoin her class or group.

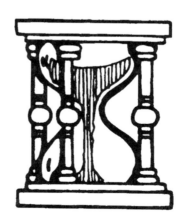

CHAPTER 6

The Needs of Older Children with FAS/FAE

Basic Living Skills

Techniques

☐ Line Up the Cards

☐ The Breakfast Club

☐ Cooking Meals

☐ Taking Care of Hygienic Needs

☐ Handling Money

☐ Telling Time

☐ Chores

While it is good to encourage academic learning in children with FAS/FAE, it is just as important that they learn basic living skills on a daily basis. It can't be taken for granted that as they grow older they will just naturally learn how to cook nutritious meals, eat regularly, bathe daily, dress appropriately, take care of their possessions,

115

clean up after themselves, handle money responsibly, show up for work and appointments on time, etc. They need to be taught these skills over and over again. In many cases, even when they become adults they will still need guidelines and supervision.

Line Up the Cards

Appropriate for Ages: 5 to adolescent.

Materials Needed: 3×5 index cards, marking pens.

Goal: To identify the order of things in a child's day.

Follow-up: Frequent repetition.

Setting: One-on-one or group.

Have the child identify what responsibilities she has in the course of a day, breaking the day into three parts and describing what is expected of her during each of those parts. For instance, the parts might include Before School, After School, and Evening. Depending on how much the child is capable of processing at once, have her choose four to six 3×5 cards that she will draw pictures or symbols on, that depict what her responsibilities are. Her "Before School" cards might have pictures or symbols that represent: eating breakfast, getting dressed, making bed, brushing teeth, combing hair, walking to the bus stop for school.

The idea is to help the child remember the order of things in her routine. Each card should be numbered, according to where the activity falls in the order of her day. It generally isn't necessary to go into detail regarding time spent at school, since school has its own routine and is usually consistent, but other times of the day can present problems. If the child is new to a school, having the "School" cards may be beneficial.

This exercise also works well for an adolescent who is starting a job. Having visuals that remind him of the steps involved in his getting to work, doing his job, and returning from work, is very helpful and contributes to keeping him "on track."

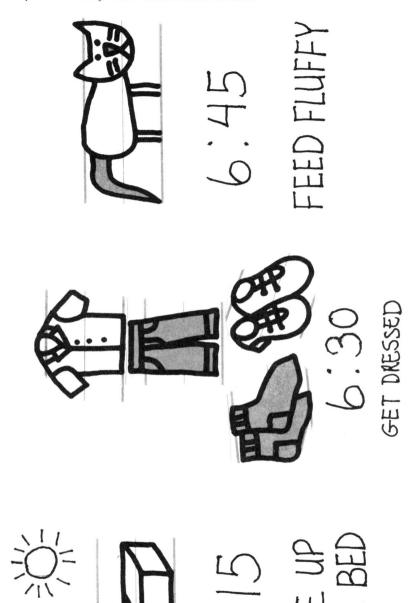

6:45 FEED FLUFFY

6:30 GET DRESSED

6:15 WAKE UP MAKE BED

7:30
HOMEWORK
BY FRONT DOOR

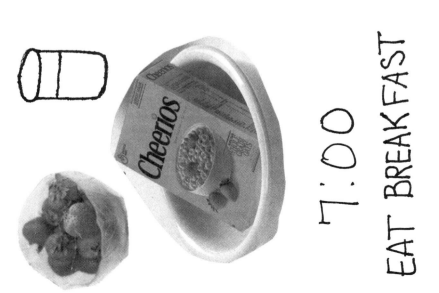

7:00
EAT BREAKFAST

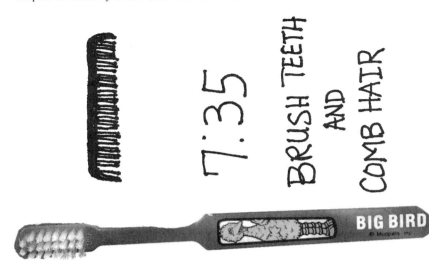

7:35

BRUSH TEETH AND COMB HAIR

BIG BIRD
© Muppets Inc

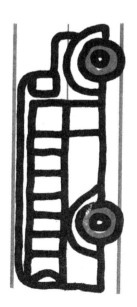

8:00

CATCH SCHOOL BUS

Another way to do this exercise (especially with older children) is to have them make a collage of their day, with the events being in sequence and numbered the way the cards would be.

The Breakfast Club

One special education teacher has created what she calls "The Breakfast Club." Every Friday morning she brings to school a variety of foods to prepare. She also brings her electric skillet and the utensils needed for the cooking project. Her students are assigned jobs to do, which include helping with the cooking, setting the table, and cleaning up after the meal is over.

Needless to say, these students look forward to Fridays! They learn by participating, hands-on, and they have a good time. In addition to teaching them meal preparation, their teacher also coaches them on hygiene (washing their hands, wiping their mouths during the meal, cleaning up after themselves) and etiquette (setting the table, using the right silverware, having good table manners). The Breakfast Club is a very valuable part of the teacher's curriculum and the lessons learned on Friday by these children will serve them well throughout their lives.

Cooking a Meal

Make the child with FAS/FAE the "chef" of a simple meal. Include him in the planning of what he will be cooking. Then make a list of what steps will be necessary in the fixing of the meal. Encourage him to focus on just one step at a time (so that he doesn't become overwhelmed). Let him know that you are there to help him with whatever he finds difficult but let him do as much of the work as possible.

Once he "masters" fixing the meal several times, suggest that he try something new to cook. For items that the child is likely to cook often, you may want to make a time chart. To do this:

❑ Paste a picture of each item on a piece of tagboard. Assign a color to it (chocolate brownies/brown)

❑ Write the number of minutes required for cooking the item next to the picture. Use the "assigned" color to write out the minutes

❑ Then put corresponding color dots or marks next to the number minute lines on a white, wind-up kitchen timer (colored tape, dots or model paint can be used to make the marks). This lets the child know how many minutes are needed to cook which items

Taking Care of Hygienic Needs

Remembering to attend to their basic hygienic needs is not often a priority of children with FAS/FAE. In fact, it can sometimes become quite a challenge to get them to bathe, brush their teeth, comb their hair, etc. Making a game out of their maintaining cleanliness seems to be the approach that works best.

One mother shared that she "races" her FAS son to get him to get ready for school in the morning. She bets him that she can have his lunch made before he has his teeth brushed, face washed, and hair combed. Most of the time, her method works. With some children, direct supervision is necessary.

Another mother made a sticker chart for hygienic needs alone. Her daughter earned points for both morning and bedtime cleanliness and at the end of the week got a sticker. Four stickers earned her a prize.

You might want to make up an ongoing story about a child who always remembers to bathe, brush his teeth, comb his hair, clean his ears, etc. Whenever you want a younger child with FAS/FAE to do any of these same things you can say, "Remember what Christopher Clean does? Let's pretend we are right beside him, doing everything he does."

Repetition is the key in teaching children with FAS/FAE about personal hygiene. Intellectually they may not understand why it is important to be clean, but if you can make it a fun experience with lots of positive reinforcement, they are more apt to follow through with what you want them to do.

Handling Money

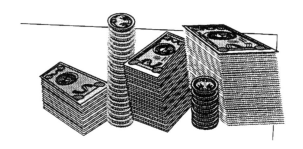

Teaching children with FAS/FAE how to handle their money responsibly is another challenge. It is sometimes hard for them to grasp that coins amount to dollars and vice versa. It may help if you take a small glass or clear container and tell the child with FAS/FAE that the glass represents a dollar bill. Then fill the glass with coins that equal a dollar so they can see how this is so. Explain to her that two containers filled with the same amount of change equals two dollars, etc. Then take her to the store to buy two one-dollar items. Have her pay for one with a dollar bill and the other with the change from the one-dollar container. This will help her grasp the concept you are trying to teach her.

You may also want to set up a store in your home or at school so the child can practice buying things and receiving and counting change. Again, some children with FAS/FAE may be better at this than others. For those who have difficulty, keep the exchanges simple and repeat them over and over.

One mother was concerned about her seventeen-year-old son's carelessness regarding money so she decided to give him a daily allowance in coins. Each day she gave him a little less money. Finally, after several days, he realized that he was being short-changed and he confronted his mother about it. She was then able to convince him that he needed to be more responsible about keeping track of his money.

If possible, open a bank account for the child with FAS/FAE. Let her make regular deposits and help her keep her bank book up to date. For saving money before taking it in to make a deposit, a clear bank with individual slots for quarters, dimes, nickels and pennies is excellent. It shows how many coins add up to what amount of money. The visual image is good for the child with FAS/FAE to have.

Telling Time

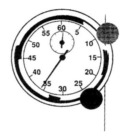

We've already mentioned how digital clocks work best for children with FAS/FAE because reading them does not require abstract thinking. The mother of a nine-year-old boy with FAS discovered that her son thought of time as something spatially linear, rather than in terms of seconds, minutes, and hours. One day when she asked him how long an assembly at school had been, he took several steps backward and said, "About this long."

Realizing that her son was showing her how he perceived time, she got out a pair of scissors and some paper and cut strips of paper of different sizes. She then asked him to choose the pieces that best represented how long his favorite TV show was, how long it took him to walk to his best friend's house, how long he spent brushing his teeth in the morning, etc. Her recognition of her son's unique way of perceiving time and then her willingness to "translate" it for him by cutting paper into shapes gave them both a common "language" to use when it was necessary to discuss time.

It is also wise not to tell the child with FAS/FAE about upcoming events too far in advance. Because hours and minutes may be meaningless to him, you will get asked dozens of times, "Is it time now?" Wait until it is certain that the change or event is going to take place, and then tell the child several minutes before. This will reduce the stress for both of you.

Chores

Assigning simple chores for a child with FAS/FAE is important. Of course, you must take into consideration the child's emotional and intellectual development. It is also beneficial if the assigned chores are ones he will succeed at most of the time. Reminding and even supervising him will probably be necessary but each time he completes a chore and is acknowledged for doing so, his self-esteem grows.

Making a chore chart with him is helpful. He needs to know exactly what is expected of him and when. Keep changes in the routine to a minimum (for instance, rotating chores every week with other family members or students might be too confusing for the child with FAS/FAE). Introducing one chore at a time and giving him the opportunity to master it before adding another one is what tends to work best.

As the child gets into adolescence, the way he follows through with chores may indicate how he will perform on the job. The child with FAS/FAE often starts something with great enthusiasm, only to lose interest in it or become distracted by something else in a short period of time. Encouraging the child to "stick with" a chore until it is completed and then praising him for doing so is an approach that works well.

	Monday	Tuesday					
EMPTY GARBAGE Monday, Thursday, Saturday	X		X		X	X	
FEED JASPER DAILY	X	X	X	X	X	X	X
LOAD DISHWASHER After Dinner Tuesday and Thursday		X	X				

Social Skills

❏ The Spotlight

❏ Puppet Show

Learning social skills is an important piece of learning basic living skills. The child with FAS/FAE remains emotionally immature even as she develops an adult body. In our society there is little tolerance for an adult who often acts like a child. We must begin teaching the child with FAS/FAE social skills when she is very young. She needs to learn to respect the boundaries of others and to express her feelings in appropriate ways.

The Spotlight

Appropriate for Ages: 3 to adult.

Materials Needed: A flashlight, hula hoop, masking tape or long piece of string.

Goal: To encircle the child/adolescent/adult so that she can visually see the boundary that allows her personal space.

Follow-up: To discuss the importance of her maintaining her own personal space (unless she invites someone else into it) and also respecting the personal space of others.

Setting: One-on-one or in a group.

One technique that is used to teach about respecting boundaries is The Spotlight. Shine the beam of a large flashlight on the floor and tell the child with FAS/FAE to step into the middle of it. Then you can say, "This is your very own spotlight—your personal boundary. You get to decide who steps inside of it and who stays on the outside."

Then you can explain that everyone has their own boundary surrounding them, even though it isn't something that others can see. Stress that it is important for her to respect the boundaries of others. She can do this by not getting too close or touching someone without their permission, not talking out of turn, and not taking other people's things unless she is told that she can do so.

Another way to illustrate the boundary concept is to use string or tape to encircle the child with FAS/FAE, and then refer to the circle as their boundary. One mother called her boundary her "halo" and when her child moved in too close, she would say, "You are breaking my halo."

Expressing her feelings in appropriate ways is also something we must constantly help the child with FAS/FAE learn to do. As adults, we may often have to act as the child's "thermostat" when her frustration level rises and she begins to act out. Helping the child with FAS/FAE maintain her emotional balance requires strength, patience, and a positive attitude. She needs adult role models who are able to acknowledge and express their feelings appropriately, so she can learn how to do the same.

Puppet Show

Appropriate for Ages: 6 to adolescent.

Materials Needed: A variety of hand and/or finger puppets as well as other "props" for puppet show, depending on the topic. (For instance, cigarettes, if the topic is smoking versus not smoking, or a purse if you are teaching not stealing, etc.)

Goal: To let group members act out situations where they need to use appropriate social skills.

Follow-up: To discuss the pros and cons of their actions and decisions.

Setting: Excellent for using in group settings.

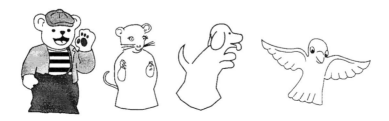

Divide the group into teams. Give each team a topic to act out before the other group members. Tell them to first act out the inappropriate behavior, and then have them demonstrate the use of appropriate behavior in the same situation.

Wise Choices

❑ Plan A / Plan B

❑ The Fish Bowl

❑ The Y Game

❑ Slippery Situations

Often the child with FAS/FAE has poor judgment, low impulse control, and a hard time distinguishing right from wrong. This makes it difficult for him to make wise choices, but whenever he does, it is important that he receive lots of praise. Something that works well is setting up a situation for him where he gets to make a choice (under your supervision). Then you can immediately say, "I see you've chosen to do this," or "I like the choice you've made. It's a good one," making him aware of his ability to choose and letting him know that you support his choice. When he moves on to something else, you can then say, "I see you've made a choice to do something else. I'm proud of you," etc.

It is easy for us to focus on the shortcomings of children with FAS/FAE. What they need to see and hear is that we notice the things that they do right.

Plan A / Plan B

Appropriate for Ages: 10 to adult.

Materials Needed: A large piece of paper or tagboard, colored pens.

Goal: To encourage the child/adolescent/adult to consider two different options.

Follow-up: To discuss the contents of his goal pyramids and how he plans to attain each step he has identified.

Setting: One-on-one or can be used as a group exercise if each participant is given some individual attention.

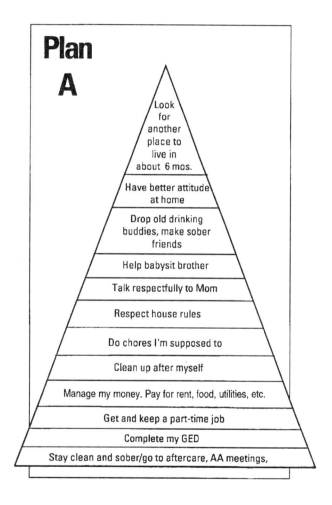

It is not uncommon for the child with FAS/FAE to be very stubborn and resist making choices or changes. Likewise, he may resist choices that are made for him. The Plan A / Plan B approach is often effective because it helps

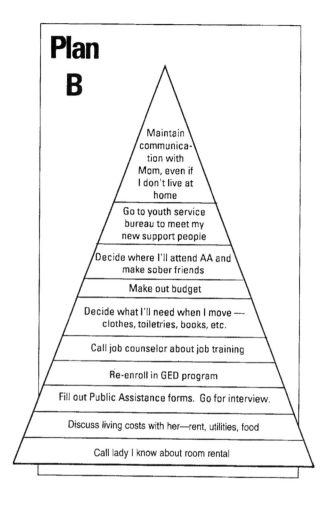

Plan B

Maintain communica-tion with Mom, even if I don't live at home

Go to youth service bureau to meet my new support people

Decide where I'll attend AA and make sober friends

Make out budget

Decide what I'll need when I move — clothes, toiletries, books, etc.

Call job counselor about job training

Re-enroll in GED program

Fill out Public Assistance forms. Go for interview.

Discuss living costs with her—rent, utilities, food

Call lady I know about room rental

avoid power struggles and makes the child more aware of his options. For example: When I was a case manager at a treatment center for chemically dependent adolescents, I had an FAE child who turned 18 while he was in treatment. There were many family problems and during a counseling session with the boy (John) and his mother, she announced that when he graduated from treatment, she didn't want him to come back home. She was adamant about this and he was just as adamant about refusing to believe her.

For two weeks I tried to help John break through his resistance. He needed to start taking the necessary steps to find a place to live. He also needed to apply for public assistance and enroll in a GED program. There was so much I wanted to help him with, but he was hurt and overwhelmed and couldn't see his options. He had a plan that he wanted to cling to and that was to go back home and "have everything be okay." It was at this point that I came up with the Plan A / Plan B technique.

Plan A is the one the child insists upon. It is important that you honor that. Resisting it and telling him that "it will never work, it's a ridiculous plan, my plan is much more sensible," etc., will only cause the child to resist you even more. Instead, you might say something like "I see that you really believe in your plan. Good for you. Not everybody can be so sure of themselves. Let's call your plan Plan A. Now, pretend you are a football coach who wants his team to win a very important game. He has his players practice and practice a certain way because he is sure that he knows just how they can beat the other team. He has a 'game plan' that we will call Plan A. The night of the game arrives and the coach says to his team, 'Remember to follow our game plan.' The team nods and heads for the field. All through the first half they stick to the game plan, just as they practiced it. At halftime, though, they are behind, 20 to 0. What do you think the coach is going to do? Do you think that he will stick to the game plan—to Plan A?"

Go on to say that the coach quickly shifted to a different game plan because he realized that Plan A just wasn't going to work. Then say, "Maybe your Plan A will work just fine, but it is always good to have a Plan B, as well. I want to see you succeed. Let's go over your Plan A and make sure I understand it, okay? Then, if you want, we can talk about a Plan B."

Most of the time the child is open to trying this if you honor his original plan. To go on with the exercise, draw two large triangles (poster-size). Label one Plan A and the other Plan B. At the top of each triangle, write the word "Goal."

Then, beginning with Plan A, ask the child to tell you what steps he must take to reach his Plan A goal. For instance, John's steps included:

1. Stay clean and sober/go to Aftercare AA meetings, etc.

2. Complete my GED

3. Get and keep a part-time job

4. Manage my money. Give Mom money for rent, food and utilities. Put some money into a savings account

5. Clean up after myself

6. Do chores that Mom wants me to

7. Respect house rules

8. Talk respectfully to Mom

9. Help babysit my younger brother

10. Drop old drinking buddies and make new friends who are clean and sober

11. Have a better attitude at home

12. Look for another place to live in about 6 months (when I'm more sure of myself)

We listed each step inside his pyramid, beginning with #1 and ending with #12 as the goal at the top.

Once the child completes his first pyramid, praise him for doing such a good job, no matter how simplistic (or unrealistic) his plan may be. This praise is important because it is what will motivate him to make a Plan B. Another important piece is to let the child spend time with his Plan A before going right into Plan B. After all, Plan A was his idea and letting him have several minutes with it shows him that you respect his investment in his original plan.

The process for making Plan B is the same. It may, however, require more assistance on your part because it introduces options to the child that he isn't aware of and might need time to consider. John's Plan B included:

1. Call lady I know who once said I could rent a room in her house

2. Discuss living costs with her—rent, food, utilities

3. Fill out forms for public assistance and go for an interview

4. Re-enroll in the GED program I was in

5. Call a job counselor at youth service bureau about a possible part-time job or job training

6. Make a list of items I'll need when I move—clothes, toiletries, books, etc.

7. Make out a budget

8. Decide where I'll attend AA/NA meetings—get a sponsor, make new, sober friends, drop drinking buddies

9. Go with Diane to youth service bureau to meet my new case manager, GED teacher and job counselor

10. Maintain communication with Mom even if I don't live at home

Once John saw his Plan B in writing, something began to change for him. He became less resistant to the idea of living on his own. In fact, with guidelines to follow, he began to like the idea of Plan B, after all.

After the child has completed both pyramids, encourage him to put them up on a wall where he can look at them frequently, especially before he goes to sleep at night, and when he wakes up in the morning. The object is to help the child become so familiar with all of his options that he will feel safer with the necessary changes he may have to make.

The Plan A / Plan B technique is very effective when major changes have to be made (such as changing schools, looking for a job, behavior modification, etc.) and the child has time to get used to all of his options. It can also be used as a verbal exercise when there isn't much time, such as during a conflict with another person. With a situation like this, you may say, "Plan A can be that you stay angry at

Suzy or Plan B can be that you use the crib mattress or bats and balloon to get your energy out. Then, once you do that, you might feel more like talking things over with her and settling your argument."

In John's case, he became so empowered by learning about Plan A / Plan B that he was able to apply the technique to the short-term situations that came up for him during the rest of his stay in treatment. He also decided to take the steps he listed on his Plan B pyramid and was successful in finding a room to rent, enrolling in a GED program, and working his 12-step program to remain clean and sober. He was fortunate that he had a number of people who were there to "watch out for him," mainly his landlady, who included him in the family and helped him with money management.

John had a high enough I.Q. to really think through all the steps on both of the pyramids. Some children with FAS/FAE may not be able to be as detailed or follow through with such enthusiasm. You will have to be sensitive to the capabilities of each child you try this technique with, and let them set the pace, especially when you are working on plans that are long-term.

The Fish Bowl

Appropriate for Ages: 6 to Adolescent.

Materials Needed: Fish bowl, slips of paper, marking pens.

Goal: To teach appropriate decision-making and social skills.

Follow-up: Repeat this exercise often.

Setting: One-on-one, group.

After a discussion with the child or group about some basic, appropriate social skills, write short descriptions of various social situations on slips of paper. Put the slips of paper in the fish bowl and let the child (or in a group setting, one child at a time), reach into the bowl and pull out one of the slips of paper. The child will then read the situation out loud (an adult may have to do the reading if the child can't read) and describe how he would handle that situation. Or, the child will read the situation and other group members can describe how they might handle the situation.

The social situations written on the slips of paper should be age-appropriate. Some topics for younger children might include:

❑ When I am standing in line at school I should keep my hands to myself because . . .

❑ When someone in my class is having a turn at show-and-tell I need to keep quiet because . . .

❑ If I am walking home and a person I have not met before offers me a ride, I should . . .

Topics for older children (adolescents) might include:

❑ When I see my mother's car keys on the table and I want to try driving while she is taking a nap I should . . .

❑ When the kids at school ask me to play a joke on the science teacher, I need to tell them . . .

❑ When somebody I really want to be friends with asks me to sneak him some beer out of the mini-market while he talks to the cashier, I should . . .

The individual working with the child or group will know what issues need to be dealt with and should include them, accordingly. Some younger children may be quite "street wise" so questions that are asked of the adolescents might also be appropriate for these younger children.

The Y Game

Appropriate for Ages: 5 to adolescent.

Materials Needed: Blackboard and chalk.

Goal: To help children learn to make the right decisions.

Follow-up: Repeat exercise often.

Setting: One-on-one or group.

Draw a large Y on the blackboard. Explain that one branch of the Y represents The Little Green Guy and the other branch represents the Stronger Self (who doesn't want to get into trouble). Then describe a situation and ask the child or group what the Little Green Guy would do in it and then what the Stronger Self would do. Encourage the child or group members to share some real-life situations that they have been confronted with and use those in the Y Game, as well.

Slippery Situations

Appropriate for Ages: 8 to adolescent.

Materials Needed: Colored paper, vaseline, spoon.

Goal: For child to identify what "slippery situations" are.

Follow-up: Discussion of slippery situations and how to avoid them.

Setting: One-on-one or group.

In chemical dependency treatment settings we call situations which are unhealthy and likely to cause trouble "slippery situations." Because children with FAS/FAE are often very tactile, this exercise is especially effective in helping them remember slippery situations.

You might want to use some of the same examples of life situations that were used in the Fish Bowl and Y Games. Discuss them with the child or group and then ask them to choose one that they particularly relate to and draw it on the colored paper with the spoonful of vaseline you have given them. If it is a group exercise, have each person hold his drawing up and explain it to you and the other group members. Making a book of slippery situations is also effective. For a book, however, you would want to use marking pens or crayons, rather than vaseline.

CHAPTER 7

For Parents and Counselors with Adolescents and Adults with FAS/FAE

Finding Jobs

Finding vocations for adolescents and adults with FAS/FAE can be challenging. Many parents say that their adolescents with FAS/FAE may find jobs, but they then have trouble keeping them. This is often due to their failing to show up for work or not performing their duties consistently.

If you have an adolescent with FAS/FAE you want to find work for, spend time determining what his strengths and interests are. Many adolescents with FAS/FAE are artistic, musical, athletic, mechanical, enjoy cooking, and are good conversationalists. If they are nonviolent, they can also be very good with young children, animals, and the elderly.

It is important to keep in mind that his job environment should be one where there is structure, order and routine, and where he will be supervised by adults who are patient and understand his limitations. He may need someone to take him to and from work to make sure he gets to his destination. Often, the adolescent or adult with FAS/FAE

137

gets distracted on his way to work and decides to go some-where else instead. He acts on impulse and doesn't think about the consequences.

Eventually, we hope to establish vocational schools where adolescents and adults with FAS/FAE will receive specialized training based on their strengths, and then placed in special job centers where they are supervised closely and given lots of positive reinforcement for the work they accomplish.

Chemical Dependency Risks

Children with FAS/FAE are high risk for becoming chemi-cally dependent. Studies show that alcoholism is a disease that is passed on from generation to generation whether the child lives with the alcoholic parent(s) or not. It is also a fact that most adolescents who drink tend to use other drugs, as well.

Early prevention is so important in our work with chil-dren with FAS/FAE. We must regularly remind them that drinking and using other drugs can cause them many prob-lems, and that pregnant women should never drink or use other drugs. We need to show them alternative ways of hav-ing fun, dealing with their feelings and being accepted by others. Too often their desire to "fit in" coupled with their poor judgment can lead them to drinking and other chemi-cal abuse. We especially need to supervise them as they get older because they are exposed to so many more negative influences.

If a child with FAS/FAE starts drinking alcohol (and using other drugs) on a regular basis, it is quite possible that she will become chemically dependent within a year or so (or even sooner). In such cases, it is wise to get the child into a treatment center so that she receives the help she will need to stop drinking and using other drugs. It is often hard for people in our society to believe that a child can become an alcoholic at an early age, but it does happen. In order for children and adolescents with FAS/FAE to get the kind of intervention they need, I would recommend inpatient treatment rather than outpatient treatment for them.

Inpatient Treatment

In many ways, adolescents (and adults) with FAS/FAE who are in inpatient treatment centers thrive because of the structure, order, and routine of the facility, as well as from the attention they get from their case managers and other counselors. However, if they are expected to grasp the meaning of the twelve steps, do written assignments, and act socially appropriate, they may not be able to "keep up" with their peers.

As in the school setting, it is very important for treatment center staff to be educated about fetal alcohol syndrome. Each client with FAS/FAE should be seen as a unique individual who may have special needs that the other clients at the same center may not have. His treatment plan should have realistic goals for him to meet, based on his own personal strengths, rather than what is expected from "the norm."

Clients with FAS/FAE will need close supervision. The areas where they may have problems include:

❑ Interacting socially with other clients and staff in appropriate ways

❑ Being able to stay focused during lectures and therapy groups (and grasping and retaining the information being discussed)

❑ Understanding and completing written assignments

❑ Following directions that are given too quickly and/or are not supervised

❑ Taking care of basic hygienic needs

❑ Remembering to do assigned chores

Behavior problems may include:

❑ Lying

❑ Stealing

❑ Anger Outbursts

❑ Sexual Acting Out

❑ Setting Fires

❑ Destroying Property

❑ Running Away

Knowing the History

Knowing the history of the child with FAS/FAE who is in treatment is imperative. During the intake, questions about family history and chemical use are routinely asked, but it is also important to find out about medical, behavioral, and academic history.

As a case manager, you may see behaviors surface in your client that have not been reported by the parents. It is your job to acknowledge these behaviors and along with others on staff, determine how to best deal with them. The advantages of having these clients in treatment are:

❑ They have twenty-four hour supervision

❑ Behaviors and needs are identified and efforts are made to manage the behaviors and meet the needs

❑ Clients get structure, order, and routine

❑ Other family members are involved in the treatment process

❑ Clients are educated about chemical dependency, behavior management, and appropriate social skills

Clients with FAS/FAE will most likely need lots of guidance throughout the treatment stay. As in the school setting, too much information coming at them at once, sudden changes in the routine, and exposure to lots of stimulation can be very upsetting to them. They also may be ostracized or victimized by the other clients.

Being able to instill in them the dangers of alcohol and other drug use may also be a challenge. Some may be able to grasp the concept better than others. It will depend upon how well they retain information and are able to control their impulses. If they are taught with visuals and concrete examples, they may be able to remember better. Allow them to take an active part in the learning. Techniques that often work well are:

❑ Providing puppets and other props for them to do skits (about family dynamics, feelings, drug-using behavior, etc.)

❑ Supervised art work, e.g., drawing, painting, making collages, working with clay, mask-making, etc.

❑ Physical activity (especially to manage anger and release energy in appropriate ways), e.g., shooting baskets, running laps, lifting weights, jumping rope, doing push-ups, dancing, etc.

❑ Music (one child with FAS/FAE did his homework by writing rap songs—the answers were in the lyrics)

❑ Meditation

As I have said before, many of the techniques I use with younger children with FAS/FAE also work well with adolescents and adults. You may want to use the same prop, but change the message to apply more specifically to a situation. For instance, when I work with chemically dependent clients I refer to "The Little Green Guy" as "The Addictive Self" who encourages the person who is trying to stay clean and sober to go ahead and use anyway. Slugs represent how a person feels inside when he relapses. The Goal Pyramids are effective not only in planning aftercare, but also in comparing choosing a life of chemical dependency versus staying clean and sober.

Planning Aftercare

Having a clear, realistic aftercare plan is essential for clients with FAS/FAE. As in the treatment plan, goals must be realistic and based on what the client is capable of, emotionally, physically and intellectually, rather than what we would like him to be able to accomplish. Family support is key in the success of the chemically dependent person with FAS/FAE. There needs to be strong supervision to help the client stay off alcohol and other drugs. Enlisting the help and support of others outside the family is also wise. The client will need a patient, caring sponsor and a chemical dependency counselor who both understand FAS/FAE. There may also be a need for a job counselor and a GED instructor or tutor. Clients with FAS/FAE who are getting out of treatment have many of the same challenges before them that clients without FAS/FAE do. They are also extremely vulnerable to relapse because of their low impulse control, poor judgment and inability to distinguish right from wrong. In treatment they are closely supervised and can count on the consistency of their environment. The "real world" is a much different place. As one mother put it, "They need to be protected from society and society needs to be protected from them."

In the right treatment facility, clients with FAS/FAE are safe and can function fairly well. As a society, we need to provide more settings like this for our children, adolescents and adults who have FAS/FAE. They may not necessarily be for treating chemical dependency, but the model is a good one and can certainly reinforce prevention.

Children with FAS/FAE and the Law

Our legal system is set up with the assumption that violators of the law can distinguish right from wrong and can also learn from their mistakes. If a law is broken, a punishment is assigned. Usually, a young offender must break the law a number of times before strong intervention takes place.

Often, the penalty is for the young offender to do community service. Being assigned community service may just be another set-up for failure for a child with FAS/FAE. He may end up getting into even more trouble, or being criticized for not following through on what he is supposed to do. In a detention center or jail, he can fall in with teens who are a bad influence on him. On the other hand, if he is released to the custody of his parents and he is out of control, his parents may not know what to do with him. He can cause quite a bit of uproar within the family.

Our judicial system needs to learn more about FAS/FAE. Children with FAS/FAE need to be held accountable for their inappropriate behaviors, but believing that they will eventually understand right from wrong by being punished is unrealistic. Children with FAS/FAE who get into trouble with the law should not be treated as "normal" children. Instead, our society needs to establish group homes where these children can be closely monitored and guided in leading productive lives based on their individual abilities. (See article by Dr. Lew Abrams in *Articles* section.)

Because we are only just beginning to understand the special needs of children with FAS/FAE, few group homes exist that are specifically set up for them. You may want to check with the Department of Juvenile Justice or the Department of Social and Health Services in your state, to see what group homes are presently available.

Birth Control

As they approach puberty, birth control for children with FAS/FAE becomes an important issue. Their sex drive is normal but, again, their poor judgment and their lack of impulse control causes them to engage in sexual activity without considering the consequences. They can also be made victims by others who use them for sex or encourage them to be promiscuous. When alcohol and other drugs are involved, the risks of pregnancy and disease become even higher.

Prevention may include educating children with FAS/FAE about sex and birth control, but monitoring them is even more important. It is unrealistic to expect that they won't want to try sex simply because they've been told not to. Their focus is on the moment, and if they feel like having sex or someone instructs them to do so, it is very likely that they will.

Parents struggle with their many concerns regarding puberty and birth control. What to do becomes their responsibility, rather than the responsibility of their adolescents with FAS/FAE. For now, parents have no "set" answers, but they do have other parents of children with FAS/FAE to turn to for ideas and emotional support.

In Summary

Although fetal alcohol syndrome and fetal alcohol effects have been around for centuries, we have only just begun to address the needs of children with FAS/FAE and their families. What we know is that children with FAS/FAE never outgrow their handicap, and that they need our guidance and support to help them lead the happiest, safest, most productive lives possible.

We know, too, that even though children with FAS/FAE share many common characteristics and behaviors, they are still very unique individuals with their own feelings, "spirits," and personalities. It is so important that we nurture them, not only by providing positive home and school environments but by honoring who they are as persons.

The research goes on, as do our efforts to raise the level of awareness in our society about the devastating effects that alcohol can have on the unborn. You can help by sharing what you learn about FAS/FAE with others, and by supporting legislation that will provide funding for those affected by FAS/FAE.

There are many "ups and downs" in raising, teaching, and working with children with FAS/FAE. It takes special people to deal with such special children. The good news is that now so much more information about FAS/FAE is available, support networks are growing, and the needs of children with FAS/FAE and their families are beginning to be addressed around the country.

There is still much work to be done but the commitment is there and the "troops" are growing in number. As we deal with the destruction that prenatal drinking has already caused, we can clearly see how important teaching prevention is. Reaching out to children with FAS/FAE and their families must also include reaching out to the children who are yet to be conceived. If women don't drink during pregnancy, babies with FAS/FAE won't be born. Prevention is the answer. We are the ones to carry the message.

SECTION III

ARTICLES AND OTHER RESOURCES

Diagnosing Fetal Alcohol Syndrome

by Michael Donlan, M.D.

Although Fetal Alcohol Syndrome (FAS) was not brought to the attention of the medical community until 1973, concerns about the possibility of alcohol use causing problems during pregnancy can be traced back into ancient times. In the Old Testament, an angel admonished Samson's mother: "Behold, thou shall conceive, and bear a son; and now drink no wine or strong drink" (Judges 13:17). In ancient Carthage the drinking of wine was forbidden to the bridal couple on their wedding night to help avoid the conception of defective children. In 1834 a report to the British House of Commons indicated that infants born to alcoholic mothers had a "starved, shriveled and imperfect look."

The incidence of FAS has been estimated to be 1 in 300 to 1 in 2000 live births. It is easily the leading cause of mental retardation in the western world. The cost is staggering—estimated to be $320 million per year for treatment alone . . . and this does not include institutional care. Additionally the lifetime cost of care for one FAS child has been estimated to be $1.4 million. The incidence of fetal alcohol effect (FAE) is felt to easily be double the number of cases of FAS.

The use of alcohol by mothers during pregnancy has clearly been shown to affect the physical development and the mental development of babies. However not all babies whose mothers drink during their pregnancy will have the full-blown Fetal Alcohol Syndrome.

The diagnosis of a syndrome in medicine is based upon a constellation of findings from the history and the physical examination of a person. It is similar to putting together a puzzle and trying to find pieces that fit together to make a picture. Fetal Alcohol Syndrome babies have findings based on the history and physical examination which makes it possible to identify and diagnose the condition. Fetal Alcohol Effect (FAE) is NOT a medical diagnosis but nonetheless appears to be the learning and behavioral results of the use of alcohol by a mother during pregnancy. However, babies, children and adults with FAE are not recognized clinically (i.e. on physical examination)—BUT the effects of maternal alcohol use during pregnancy are just as real. Some of the more common physical findings in children with FAS are:

1. The babies are small (both for height and weight) when they are born and they remain small throughout childhood

2. They have small head size at birth and this persists in about 28% throughout their life. The small head size is a reflection of both small brains and slow brain growth and development

3. The eyes show short palpebral fissures (the eye slits), a wide flat bridge of the nose and epicanthal folds (an extra skin fold on the inner aspect of the eyes). In the normal person who does not have FAS, if you measure from the outer corner of each eye you can divide this area up into nearly equal thirds. That is, one third for the right eye, one third for the nose and one third for the left eye. Children with FAS have an increased distance across the nose and a decreased distance for each eye slit

4. The nose appears to be short (this may become less noticeable with time)

5. The philtrum area (which is above the upper lip and below the nose) does not have the two prominent vertical ridges, but rather is flat and this area appears longer than normal

6. The vermilion border (the pink area) of the upper lip is smaller than the vermillion border of the lower lip

7. The face appears somewhat flattened and the chin is small when the person is seen on a side view. While the face and brain appear to be most severely affected by maternal alcohol use there may be developmental problems in other developing organs also

8. An increased chance that the fingers may have contractures (and not open all the way) and that the fifth (small) finger may be slightly incurved

9. There is more likely to be a single crease going across the entire palm of the hand (rather than two separate creases—neither of which goes all the way across the hand)

10. These children are more likely to be born with congenital heart disease, cleft lip and palate, strabismus (cross eyes)

11. These babies appear to have excess body hair at birth; this disappears with time

12. There may be an increased incidence of some types of cancers

13. Kidney development may be affected resulting in absent, misplaced or malformed kidneys

14. Abnormal development of the vertebral column may result in scoliosis

Women who continue to drink with each pregnancy seem to have children who will show more and more signs of their mother's drinking and the clinical expression of the Fetal Alcohol Syndrome with each subsequent pregnancy. Mothers who drink during the pregnancy are also more likely to have spontaneous abortion in the early months of the pregnancy.

The effect of the mother's drinking on the developing brain is shown by:

1. Slow motor development and mental retardation—the average IQ is 68

2. Learning disabilities

3. An inability to understand the consequences of their actions

4. Short attention span and hyperactivity

5. Behavior problems

Recently investigators at the University of Washington reported the results of FAS in Adolescents and Adults. They found that:

1. Short Stature and small head size persisted in their patients. There tended to be an increase in weight

2. The facial characteristics modified with time so there was increased growth in the chin and nose and that the diagnosis would be difficult without childhood photos

3. None of their patients were functioning independently in both housing and income

4. The average academic functioning was at early grade school level but 42% had an IQ above 70 and would not have qualified for remedial help in the school system. This is one of the BEST reasons for making a diagnosis of FAS—if a child has a MEDICAL diagnosis of a handicapping condition that child will qualify for special services in the school system

5. They tended to do poorest in mathematics and this was felt to be related to their difficulty with abstractions such as time and space, cause and effect, and generalizing from one situation to another

The amount of alcohol that can be safely consumed during pregnancy has also been evaluated, and the answer is unknown: In one study it was found that 11% of children born to mothers who drank 1 to 2 ounces of alcohol per day in only the first 3 months of the pregnancy had features consistent with FAS. This amount is equivalent to two to four beers, 8 to 16 ounces of wine or 2 to 4 ounces of liquor. Another study attempted to look at the relationship between lower birthweight of children born to mothers who drank more than 140g (two drinks per day) and found that there was a consistent lowering of birthweight in the infants of mothers who consumed this amount of alcohol. The present data also indicate that binge drinking can lead both to FAS and FAE. There is no SAFE amount of alcohol.

Ref:

"Teratology in Pediatric Practice", Seaver, L.H. and Hoyme, H. E. in *Pediatric Clinics of North America* 39 134 1992

"Recognition of the Fetal Alcohol Syndrome" Clarren, S.K. JAMA 245:2436 1981 "Fetal Alcohol Syndrome" Jones, K.L. *Pediatrics in Review* 8:122 -126 1986

"Recognition of the Fetal Alcohol Syndrome in Early Infancy" Jones, K.L. and Smith, D.W. *Lancet;* i: 999–1001 1973

"Pattern of Malformation in Offspring of Chronic Alcoholic Mothers" Jones, K.L. Smith D.W., Ulleland C.N. Streissguth, A.P. Lancet i: 1267–71 1973 Aase, *J. Personal Communication*

"Fetal Alcohol Syndrome in Adolescents and Adults" Streissguth, A.P., Aase, J.M., Clarren S.K., Randels, S.P., LaDue, R.A.. Smith, D.F. JAMA265, 1961, 1991

"Alcohol and the Fetus", Larroque, B. Int J. Epidiol 1992; 21 suppl l:S8–16 "The Effects of Moderate Alcohol Consumption During Pregnancy on Fetal Growth and Morphogenesis" Hanson, J.W., Steissguth, A.P., Smith, D.W. *J. Pediatr* 92: 457, 1978

*M*eeting the Needs of Northwest Native Youth Challenged by Fetal Alcohol Syndrome

by Lew Abrams, M.D.

Background

American Indian tribes across the nation have begun to recognize that Fetal Alcohol Syndrome (FAS) is one of the most serious consequences associated with the alcohol abuse that plagues many of the men, women, and young people in their communities. While the nationwide FAS incidence estimate of 1 in 750 live births indicates that this condition is not a uniquely Native American problem, FAS rates as high as 1 in 8 births documented in some Indian communities suggest the need for immediate, culturally relevant prevention and intervention programs. Although FAS education and prevention programs are becoming increasingly available, services for Indian people already living with FAS remain virtually nonexistent. In many tribal communities, children exposed to alcohol in utero remain essentially undiagnosed, at least in part because no services are available once a diagnosis has been determined. Thus, it is likely that undiagnosed FAS accounts for a portion of the repeated academic, social, behavioral and legal problems experienced by some of the young people in Indian communities.

While FAS affected children require a great deal of attention and special care during infancy and childhood, in adolescence their behavior becomes even more difficult to manage. Due to the poor judgment, impulsivity, anger outbursts, substance abuse, legal violations, academic delays, unprotected intercourse, inappropriate sexual behavior, and lack of social skills they often exhibit, adolescents and young adults with FAS are rarely able to maintain an adequate level of adjustment in home, school, or work settings. The result is that many young people with FAS either fail, drop out, or are expelled from school and are unable to maintain employment. They often fall into illegal activities and spend time in juvenile detention or jail. Their repeated acting out and failure to learn from consequences often leaves parents, foster parents or other caretakers searching for an out-of-home placement or day treatment program that can provide the structure they need. *The Northwest Native Youth FAS Networking and Planning Group is developing a comprehensive treatment, education, and vocational rehabilitation program tailored to the specific needs of American Indian adolescents and young adults challenged by Fetal Alcohol Syndrome.*

Overview

Because of the variety of needs and wide range of functioning observed in this population, a coordinated, multidisciplinary, individualized program is required. In the initial phase, a day treatment program will be developed and later, as funds allow, a residential treatment center will be established. Long range plans include combining this program with an Elders Housing Complex in order to create a multigenerational healing community. The service population will be American Indian males and females aged 12 to 21 years who are diagnosed with FAS. Referrals will be made by tribal health staff, the courts, DSHS, urban Indian programs, substance abuse treatment facilities, and the University of Washington FAS screening and diagnostic clinic. The program will be centrally located in the Puget Sound Region of Washington State in order to allow as many participants as possible to reach the program sites from their home communities. (The exact location for the program has yet to be determined.) Once the residential portion of the program is in place, youth who live beyond commuting distance or who do not have a viable living arrangement will be included. Assessment of potential participants will be available through Anne Streissguth, Ph.D. and Sterling Clarren, M.D., two of the world's leading experts on FAS, at the University of Washington in Seattle.

The program will seek to ensure the physical, mental, emotional, and spiritual well being of participants through a series of services designed to enhance their ability to function at the highest possible level. In addition to state-of-the-art health, special education, and substance abuse services adapted to meet the needs of each participant, activities emphasizing Indian culture and spirituality will be included in all aspects of the program. Basic living skills and mental health services will be integrated into hands-on vocational and experiential education activities, including therapeutic horsemanship, wilderness camping, canoeing, and ropes courses. Spiritual development will be encouraged by visiting religious leaders and medicine people from a variety of traditions who will lead talking circles, sweat lodges, and prayer ceremonies for interested participants. Vocational rehabilitation will take place in cottage industries set up by Native elders or others skilled in basketry, woodcarving, beadwork, drum and rattle making, and smoked salmon. An apprenticeship model will be utilized to provide participants with close supervision and to encourage the development of mentor relationships. As participants are ready, vocational training in community work settings will be arranged, facilitated by on-site job coaches who will ensure that participants receive the individualized support they need to make a satisfactory adjustment. *The overall goal of this program will be to help participants to develop practical independent living and work skills that will enable them to make a contribution to their home communities.*

The Challenge

Development of a comprehensive Native American FAS program will require the identification of substantial human and fiscal resources. Collaboration from a variety of public and private organizations will be necessary to achieve this goal. Several private foundations, such as Robert Wood Johnson, Kellogg, and Medina have been identified as potential sources of funding. Increasing tribal involvement, identifying potential sites for the program, and actively applying for grant money are the next steps.

A planning group consisting of representatives from Indian tribes and organizations, government agencies, the University of Washington, and private citizens has worked together since March of 1992 to guide the development of this program. The group is currently exploring the option of joining with an existing non-profit organization such as the United Indians of All Tribes, NW Indian College, or the Seattle Indian Health Board, rather than forming a new private non-profit corporation to carry out this program. The Seattle Indian Health Board has expressed strong interest in this possibility.

If you would like a more complete description of this proposal, or would like to make some suggestions about how or where it should be developed, please contact:

Lew Abrams, Ph.D. (206) 292–1471.

An Excerpt from Life in the FAS Lane

by Linda LaFever

One of the most difficult dilemmas we as parents and caretakers of our FAS children face is helping them to understand and accept "limits." The old "too much is never enough" adage truly applies to our kids. "How come I only get one candy bar?" "Why can't I have more quarters for the video games?" "Mom, why do we have to leave Abby's house, can't we just spend the night?" Doesn't this sound all too familiar? In the search to find a way to teach Danny "when its enough, its enough," I came up with an idea that incorporates fun and learning at the same time (the most effective strategy that seems to work in our home). We went on a Scavenger Hunt in Search of Limits. I thought about the situations that brought about the most difficulty and from that list I made little "tickets" that he was to draw out of a hat. We set aside a Saturday that was already full of errands and I explained the procedure to him. Whatever he drew out of the hat would be the first thing we were going to do. Some of the "tickets" were to "buy" things, some were to "do" things, some were to "find" an object. But ALL were limited to time and quantity.

Some of the examples were:

Find a red pickup truck.

Buy a pencil.

Play one video game.

Choose ONE of bowling or miniature golf.

Buy one candy bar.

Say the Pledge of Allegiance.

Go to McDonalds and get only one soft drink.

Find a weeping willow tree.

Select one book at the library.

Needless to say, our day was infinitely more complex than I had originally anticipated based on not knowing which "ticket" he was going to draw next in conjunction with where we were in our predetermined (by me) route. However, Danny learned that the "end of the fun" is not necessarily the "end of life as he knows it," and that other times and other places will enter his life and probably will have limits and he can learn to adjust and accept them. How far this lesson will go, I have no idea. I only know that in this age of enlightenment about FAS and what that really means to the patients and families, we are the pioneers, we are the research tool, and we are making history. Collectively we CAN make a difference in the outcome of the many lives that have been altered by no fault of their own. If WE don't make a difference, what difference does it make?

A Letter from Linda

"My name is Linda and I'm an alcoholic." I spoke those words for the very first time on October 11, 1987.

Alcoholism is medically defined as: "a chronic, progressive and potentially fatal disease," which is NOT a moral, social or psychiatric defect. I am now and have been in "remission" for over five years. One Day At A Time. My recovery, however beneficial to me, came too late for my ten-year-old-son Danny, who was conceived and born during my alcohol nightmare. Danny has Fetal Alcohol Syndrome; for Danny the nightmare will NEVER be over.

In sobriety I daily grow stronger, healthier, wiser and more capable of managing my life and embracing the future. With FAS, Danny will only grow bigger; never better. Never will he be capable of reaching the potential he would have had he not sustained organic brain damage through no fault of his own. Someday he will be an FAS adult; still misunderstood, rejected and dismissed by his peers and society in general, but, NOT BY ME. He is my child. It is for this reason that I focus my energies toward encouraging the biological family to enter sobriety and "accept the things they cannot change, change the things they can and have the wisdom to know the difference," for the sake of their child and for themselves.

At present the statistics indicate 40,000 FAS births every year in the United States with broader predictions reaching as high as 300,000 to include Fetal Alcohol Effects (FAE) which, though not clinically identifiable due to the lack of dysmorphology, is as debilitating and severe as the full syndrome.

Because the vast majority of FAS(E) children become victims of the "system" through Child Protective Services interventions (albeit necessary at times), multiple foster placements and inconsistent living arrangements, it is no wonder that their primary diagnosis is often further complicated by "Attachment Disorder" which is of itself an incredibly complex psychological impairment.

Having had the privilege as well as the opportunity of raising Danny in his birth home and seeing the result as compared to the children who have been further traumatized by the "system," it is my mission in life to encourage all substance abusing mothers (and fathers) to enter sobriety and regain control of their own lives which will benefit not only their children but themselves and their children to be.

Speaking to women in recovery programs, sharing behavior strategies out of my own day to day experience and taking anonymous telephone calls to encourage mothers into sobriety is my forte. I take the stand that it is time to stop the "tiptoe tactic" about hurting someone's feelings or insulting their integrity. Neither of these interpretations are valid as per the medical diagnosis of alcoholism. IT IS A DISEASE. No one says, "You're a diabetic, that's shameful," or "He's an epileptic, how disgraceful," or "People with chronic asthma should be ashamed." In another analogy, we would not hesitate for a moment to insist that a pregnant woman not ingest Thalidomide or perhaps arsenic! So why do we as a society in general step back in embarrassment and timidity to address the number one preventable cause of mental retardation in our nation today? Could it be perhaps we're afraid or cautious about focusing negative attention on our own (collectively) number one DRUG of choice which is not only legal but socially acceptable?

We desperately need a change in attitude as well as perspective: The most viable candidate to produce an FAS baby is the mother who already has one (or more) and halt the vicious cycle of repetition.

It is for this reason I feel it is imperative to reach the substance abusing mother with an approach of enlightenment, compassion, persuasion and diligence to encourage and facilitate recovery. It is a complicated and most intricate task but so very essential to this generation of children and the ones to follow.

In closing I would ask you to remember that from the birth mother's perspective "the dark prisons of grief and guilt for what is, or for what might have been, are all locked from the inside."

(This article is used with permission from *Iceberg* magazine.)

*C*ounseling Children with FAS/FAE and Their Families

by Diane Davis

Ever since I began working with families who have children with FAS or FAE I have become very aware of a number of key things that they need to talk about and need help with. First of all, parents ask that I explain to them just exactly what FAS or FAE is and where they can go to get more support and information. They also have a need to talk about the guilt they may feel, as well as the sense of hopelessness that sometimes overwhelms them. They have to be reminded that FAS and FAE never "go away" so that they don't continue to have unrealistic expectations of their children but learn, instead, to build on the positive things that are present.

"What can we do? How can we cope with this?," they ask. I tell them that each child and each family is unique and we must work together to shape a "program" that they can follow in their household. I also discuss their family's history—what patterns the parents have brought to their marriage and child-rearing that are generational, which of these patterns work and which do not. We discuss disciplining techniques, the importance of a "united parental front," and how family members nurture each other. I stress that the more "concrete" parents can be with their children with FAS/FAE, the better. We work on ways that they can do this.

With the children, I focus on their strengths and encourage them to talk about their feelings and frustrations. Many times they are just as overwhelmed as their parents are. They don't want to get into trouble, but they do. They wish that they could be "like the other kids," and stop causing so much distress in the family.

With one client, I talked to him about having an "On" switch and an "Off" switch. "Sometimes your "Off" switch just doesn't kick in when it is supposed to," I told him. We then drew two large switches. Under the "On" switch, we listed times when he wasn't able to do things appropriately or situations that might set him up to get into trouble. Under the "Off" switch we listed all of the times he had been able to stop himself and have more control of his actions. When he saw the two drawings and participated in making the lists underneath them, he had a greater sense of his ability to make choices that would work better for him. He put the two drawings up on his bedroom wall as constant reminders of his more positive choices.

Another boy likened his inappropriate behavior to a "runaway train." We talked about how his actions often got out of control and caused him to get into trouble. "It's like the engineer is dead and the train just keeps going. I need to learn how to bring the engineer back to life." We made lists of ways he could do this and people he could go to for help when he felt out of control. I use lots of play therapy and art therapy in my work with children and their families. Often the parents enjoy playing with my puppets and other props as much as their children do. It is their way of working through some of their own tension and a need for release.

Emotions can run high in homes where there is FAS and/or FAE to deal with. I have encouraged parents to set up a room or space in their homes where all family members can go to let their anger and frustrations out. One family bought a small trampoline, another family bought a punching bag. An old mattress or large pillows can be used for punching on, or a rubber hose and a solid object to beat it against, helps to release energy. *Everyone* needs to feel that it is okay to let their anger out in non-destructive ways. It is also important that things are talked through, as well. Often support groups are the best places for adults to learn how to do this, so that they can be positive role models for their children. The combination of a physical release followed by talking to someone who cares and is supportive, can be very powerful. For many families, these concepts are new, but they provide direction where before, there was such a feeling of hopelessness and helplessness. The "frontier" is new, but we can work together to find new ways to assist one another and reach out to others.

Reprinted with permission,
Iceberg, February 1991 issue

*L*iving with or Without an *FAS* or *FAE* Diagnosis

by Diane Davis

In 1991, I had the privilege of visiting a clinic where children with FAS/FAE are diagnosed. The particular day that I was there, a doctor was meeting with a young adolescent boy, his mother, and the social worker from the group home where the boy was living. According to his mother, her son had been a problem since birth. As an infant, he was irritable, had difficulties nursing, and was slow in his development. As he got older he became hyperactive and demanding. He constantly got into trouble at home and at school. He was unable to stay on task, was disruptive in the classroom, had poor grades, didn't seem to know the difference between right and wrong, needed lots of attention and supervision, and had very poor social skills. As a pre-adolescent his problems escalated and he got into trouble with the law. He had recently been placed in the group home because of his legal problems and his inability to obey the rules and get along in his mother's home.

"We don't know what to do about him, doctor," his mother said. "We are hoping for a diagnosis of some kind that will help us understand why he behaves the way he does and how we can better deal with him."

When the doctor asked the mother if she had used alcohol during her pregnancy she disclosed that yes, she had drunk at least a six-pack of beer daily during the nine months she was pregnant.

"I didn't know any better. Nobody told me it was wrong—that my baby might be harmed because of it. It was just my way of unwinding at the end of my workday."

Now in recovery, the mother better understands the damaging effects that alcohol had on her son and herself. However, she had only recently heard about FAS and FAE and that's what prompted her to make an appointment with this clinic.

While conversing with the mother and her son, the doctor was busy examining and measuring the boy's face. He also made note of the fact that the boy was short and underweight for his age. At the end of the exam he explained that the boy had the classic facial features of a child with FAS— eyes that were a specific size, shape, and distance apart, a flat midface, low nasal bridge, short nose, indistinct philtrum (the ridge between the nose and upperlip) and a thin upper lip. These factors, combined with the information about the mother's drinking and the boy's behavior and learning problems, enabled the doctor to give the mother a definite diagnosis that her child was/is a victim of Fetal Alcohol Syndrome.

But what about parents who have not yet been able to have their children diagnosed? Or what if there aren't enough known facts, such as in cases where children have been adopted and little is known about the natural mother, to make the diagnosis definite? Or what about adults who are just now being diagnosed as FAS or FAE—what can be done for *them?*

Because research in the field of FAS and FAE is still relatively new, we are in the very beginning stages of putting the services that are needed into place. A network is beginning to form nationwide (as well as internationally) and this is most exciting and encouraging. However, we have families who need help *now* and children and adults with FAS/FAE who deserve services for a condition they did not bring upon themselves.

What Is the Advantage of a Diagnosis?

For most, it is an answer—an explanation as to why these children and adults have acted and reacted the way they have. It serves as a starting point for letting go of old expectations and accepting the reality of how things are going to be. Once the acceptance comes, steps can be taken to formulate a new plan.

For the natural mother, it can also serve as a catalyst for committing herself to continuing her recovery work and for *forgiving herself,* as well. What was done was done, and often because of a lack of information and awareness. Families can learn from the experience and channel this learning into expanding positive parenting skills, educating others, and lobbying for more local, state and federal funds to continue the research and provide for those who have FAS and FAE. It can also motivate individuals to reach out to each other. The isolation and feelings of hopelessness can be replaced by friendship, empathy, support and the empowering of one another.

A Diagnosis for the Schools

Educators are just becoming aware of how many students with FAS/FAE are presently in their schools and how the numbers are growing. Because these children need lots of one-on-one attention, minimal stimulation and are not able to learn and retain information readily, schools are not prepared to adequately deal with them. If they don't qualify as learning disabled, attention deficit disorder, or as having a behavior disorder, they can fall through the cracks. Unfortunately, because of state and district guidelines, schools are often restricted from providing special services to students who do not have a "label" that qualifies them for a specific program.

How Do We Deal with the Non-Label Phenomenon?

We must sharpen our radar and begin to search for individuals within the school system who are open to learning more about FAS/FAE and the needs of these kinds of students and their families. Often a teacher is the first person to approach. Find out if they know anything at all about FAS/FAE—if they have attended any training or workshops about it or if they would be interested in reading articles that you might have on the subject (such as ones from *Iceberg*).

Many schools have staffing teams made up of the principal, school psychologist, school counselor, special ed teacher and several other teachers. They meet on a regular basis and discuss students who are having problems in school. Ask that your child be made a focus of concern at one of their meetings, and ask that you be allowed to be present at the meeting so you can explain about your son or daughter's possible FAS or FAE.

You may also try to start a parent group, if you know other mothers who drank during their pregnancies and are having problems with their children. Principals and school districts are apt to listen more carefully when parents band together to deliver a message and ask for more school support.

Find out what local groups you may join so that you can gain information and support and then share it with others. Educating society can begin with just one interaction that you may have with an individual who tells a few others. Since children spend so much of their years in school, the school is an excellent place to begin.

An Adult Has Been Diagnosed as FAS or FAE— Now What?

The main thing to remember is that you have a person in an adult body, whose emotional age may only be eight years old. Physically, that body may appear to be completely normal, or it can have definite malformations. The range is wide, as is true of what tasks these adults can easily perform, how much information they can retain, how well they can manage even the simplest of daily living skills, and how they respond to the world socially and emotionally. Some common factors are:

❑ Their academic skills are very limited

❑ They have poor judgment and little concept of what is right or wrong

❑ They are often victims because others take advantage of them

❑ They have little or no ability for handling money

❑ They may have a normal sex drive but little or no impulse control and a limited ability (if any) to care for a child of their own

❑ They may become depressed and isolated because so few people care to be around them

In our society, there is the expectation that adults who look "normal" will act like adults, not children. There is very little tolerance for the type of acting out that FAS/FAE adults may do. Because they are like children, these adults need primary caretakers who can look after them. They need to be protected. They need consistency and routine, especially in a job setting. They need tasks that they can succeed at and bosses and other adults who are patient and understanding.

Providing supervised social activities is also important. Often children and adults with FAS/FAE excel in art, music and certain sports. Being active provides a valuable outlet and brings fun into a life that can be frustrating and lonely.

Adequate medical/dental care is another area of importance. Just as young children don't always know that they need a doctor's attention or that it is time for a dental or eye examination, neither do adults with FAS/FAE. They need responsible others who will follow through with making appointments for them and seeing that they get to their appointments.

As I mentioned in an earlier article, there is also counseling that has just begun to become available for children with FAS/FAE and their families. Sometimes the family needs strengthening emotionally before it can begin to adapt to the changes that need to be made due to an FAS/FAE diagnosis or the suspicion that a family member is

FAS or FAE. Parents and siblings may need to open up and express their feelings, disappointments, fears and frustrations. They may need to become more educated about FAS/FAE. Children with FAS/FAE can also benefit from counseling. They can be introduced to specific, concrete ideas and ways of dealing with things. They also can respond in a positive way to the one-on-one attention and a person who can be objective and give them the emotional support they need.

A label may bring a sigh of relief because there is finally an explanation. It may make the victim or family eligible for certain monetary benefits (like SSI), or it may open new doors for special schooling and/or job opportunities. The bottom line, though, is that we know that children and adults with FAS/FAE need our love, strength, support and advocacy. We must do all we can to make continuing research possible, and to build upon the new programs that are just beginning to bud. And we need to honor our children and adults with FAS/FAE as individuals with special qualities and special needs regardless of whether they have a label or not.

Reprinted with permission,
Iceberg, July 1991 issue

*T*helma Valentine and *Her Six Special Students*

Three years ago the Chapter I aide at the elementary school where I worked, volunteered to take six little second grade boys that we suspected were drug-affected children and teach them all day long, for the last two weeks of school. She was finished with the program for her other students, so was able to devote all of her attention to these six boys, all of whom had been in lots of trouble, both academically and behaviorally, for most of the school year.

Thelma Valentine was the name of this gifted woman. Without any formal training about FAS/FAE, she knew instinctively what to do. First of all, she arranged the boys' desks in a horseshoe fashion. Her desk was between the two ends of the horseshoe so that the boys would be able to see her well and vice versa.

Thelma was very clear in letting the boys know her rules, her expectations, and what the daily routine would be. She informed them that if one student had to go to the bathroom, they would all go with him, and that they were to stay together and under her supervision at recess and at lunchtime.

Academically, she did not push them to do work that was clearly beyond their comprehension, but she expected them to do what they were capable of, and to do it well. They were then rewarded with dimestore toys or treats to eat. When they did especially well, they got to watch a video and have popcorn.

What Thelma discovered was that the boys were very responsive as long as she supervised them closely. If she just turned her back for a minute, however, most of them would not be able to stay on task. They needed her to keep them "grounded."

Thelma also realized that one of the reasons the boys had so often gotten into trouble on the playground was because they had no understanding of game rules. As a result, they would run around aimlessly and bother other students who were playing. With Thelma present to explain game rules to them and to help them learn how to play together, their harassing of other children stopped and they began to enjoy playing games with each other.

By the end of the two weeks, five of the six boys had made considerable progress in their academics, behavior, and social skills. They were smiling and feeling good about themselves, rather than hanging their heads because once again, they had gotten into trouble. The sixth boy was often tardy or absent. His family took little interest in his school-work or his emotional well-being, so consequently, he didn't do as well as the other students.

When school began the following year, four of the six boys returned. They looked for Thelma but she had transferred to another school. They told me how much she had taught them, and how well they were going to do in the coming year because of what they had learned from her. They sincerely meant what they said—I could see it in their eyes—but within two weeks, they were all sliding downhill. They needed the constant supervision that Thelma had given them, as well as the smaller sized classroom, the structure, order, and routine, and Thelma's belief in and love for them.

There are many children like the six boys Thelma taught. We know what they need from the school system. We owe them the opportunity to learn in a safe environment that is set up to meet their special needs. The impact can be very positive and rewarding. We must continue to advocate for the classrooms these children learn best in, and the teachers who have the patience, skills, and insight that Thelma had.

I *Didn't Know . . .*

by Marceil Ten Eyck, MC, CCDII

Sidney, my fifteen-year-old daughter, has Fetal Alcohol Syndrome because I drank alcohol heavily when I was pregnant with her. It didn't seem to make much difference that I didn't know the alcohol I was drinking could harm her, that my doctor suggested an occasional cocktail might be good for me, or that I had the "disease" of alcoholism and wasn't "responsible" for my behavior. My feelings of guilt, shame, and grief have still been overwhelming.

Sidney was born two-and-a-half months early and weighed two pounds, eight ounces. She spent several weeks in an intensive care preemie nursery. Her medical records included results of brain scans, a multitude of tests, procedures and comments about my visits and phone calls to the nursery. There was no mention of my drinking habits. Who would have asked a middle-class, professional woman who appeared to be successfully moving through the world, combining motherhood and a career as a Girl Scout Executive, if she had a drinking problem?

When Sidney was four years old, I was hospitalized with cirrhosis of the liver. A year later I was treated for alcoholism and have been abstinent since treatment.

When I first heard about Fetal Alcohol Syndrome, a cold, sick feeling lodged in the pit of my stomach. Sidney was six years old. However, I was able to convince myself that Sidney's small size, her immaturity (she was held back a second year in kindergarten), her difficulties with memory, and her extremely short attention span were due to her prematurity . . . "she must be slow catching up" . . . and the stress of her dad's and my divorce.

174

When Sidney started the seventh grade, a teacher friend suggested she be tested for learning disabilities because of her ups and downs in school. Despite her erratic progress and difficulties in school, she was denied testing because, "she is not two years behind in her classwork." My quest for testing led us to the Pregnancy and Health Study Clinic at the University of Washington and Dr. Sterling Clarren and Children's Hospital and Medical Center, where she was diagnosed as having Fetal Alcohol Syndrome. My response to the diagnosis was horror. Sidney's response was "what a relief."

That was two years ago. I told anyone who would listen that she was misdiagnosed. "She doesn't even look like an FAS kid . . . she is on the honor roll in school . . . she can play the piano!" At the same time I was reading everything I could find about FAS and trying to parent "as if" she had the problem. Sidney's tests at the University of Washington revealed her specific learning disabilities. Tests in hand, I went to her school counselor who has been very concerned and helpful, carefully scheduling her classes with teachers most appropriate for her learning styles. He also indicated that her diagnosis of FAS would guarantee more in depth help, should that become necessary. The diagnosis also means we, as a family, have been able to help Sidney because we understand now what she can and cannot do. I have been able to temper my expectations, which previously had been either too high or too low, depending on each conflicting report from her teachers. I am sure Sidney's many successes in junior high school have been the direct result of our family working hard with the school and now, finally accepting, coming to grips with, and coping with the realities of her Fetal Alcohol Syndrome. I think I began to accept her diagnosis about six months ago. Of course, with that acceptance came the necessity to deal with the same, guilt, grief, and pain that acceptance brought to the surface.

Since I accepted my alcoholism in 1980, a large part of my recovery has been focused on working through the shame, guilt, grief, and pain that the acceptance that "I am an alcoholic" brought. A big part of working through these feelings has occurred through sharing my story with others and with reaching out to help others whenever I could. I returned to school, obtained a Masters in Counseling degree with a special emphasis on working with chemically dependent individuals. For seven years I have been lucky to be working as a counselor and therapist for people impaired by alcoholism, drug addiction and mental illness. For three and a half years I have been the family counselor at an in-patient drug and alcohol treatment center for women.

In my search for services for children with FAS and their families, I discovered that very little was available. Consequently, I opened a private practice in October, 1990, so I could begin to be of service to other mothers who have FAS children. I hope to be able to share my story and recovery with others, to work with FAS families to help them cope with their grief, and parenting issues, and to be an advocate for them in the schools and agencies. I have discovered that both natural and adoptive parents share many of the same issues. I hope to assist in forming support groups for these parents.

I am willing and ready to speak, provide an in-service workshop, or training to any agency or group that would like to learn more about FAS/FAE.

(Reprinted with permission of the author. This article was originally written for *Iceberg.*)

*F*etal Alcohol Syndrome: A Letter from a Sixteen-Year-Old

by Sidney Helbock

When I first found out that I had the symptoms of Fetal Alcohol Syndrome I was confused and angry. I thought that I was different from everyone else and that I would be known for what I have. Since then, I have learned that the symptoms vary from individual to individual. It depends on during what stage of the pregnancy the mother drank, and the amount of alcohol consumed.

One of my symptoms is trouble understanding instructions. When a teacher shows us a certain topic, I can understand. Visual contact is a very important way of learning for me. Instructions sometimes confuse me. Following instructions is hard. When I'm asked or told to do something (like "take out the garbage") I won't understand, or the words will get mixed up in my mind.

Some other symptoms are not being able to follow oral instructions as well as written ones (example—Teacher giving assignment instructions orally—not being able to remember or follow them correctly); not hearing exactly what was said to me (example—My stepfather giving me a command to do, and not hearing him clearly, even in the same room. It's like I don't catch some words or phrases); being impulsive, doing or acting on excitement, not able to focus on reality if disaster strikes.

Most of the time I worry a lot, and make problems seem impossible to handle. When I worry, I make myself sick. At school sometimes I get sick to my stomach, or get a fever and feel awful.

These symptoms are very small compared to some symptoms I've heard of. Some people find it impossible to believe when I explain my problem, since they can't see the signs of FAS.

This letter is to help me guide myself and others. I want to help people learn about FAS, help parents who have kids who have it, and let other people who have it understand themselves better.

Sincerely,

Sidney, Age 16

(Reprinted with permission of the author. This letter was written for *Iceberg.*)

A dditional Resources

Books

Dorris, Michael (1989)
With a foreword by Louise Erdrich.
The Broken Cord
HarperCollins, New York, NY

A family's ongoing struggle with fetal alcohol syndrome (FAS), this is the true story of one American Indian child adopted from a reservation. The boy develops slowly and has a wide range of physical, behavioral, and mental problems which his adoptive father, despite all his loving efforts, cannot alleviate. Searching to understand why, he learns the hard facts of fetal alcohol syndrome. Can be purchased in paperback, $9.95, hard cover, $18.95, or inquire at your local library. Harper Collins, 10 E. 53rd St., New York, NY 10022.

Streissguth, A.P., LaDue, R.A. & Randels, S.P. (1989)
*A Manual on Adolescents and Adults with Fetal
   Alcohol Syndrome with Special Reference to
   American Indians (2nd ed.)*
Indian Health Service, Albuquerque, NM

A basic reference manual for those interested in learning more about this preventable consequence of alcohol ingestion. This manual is intended to make available in succinct form the latest information about fetal alcohol syndrome, especially as it relates to older children, adolescents and adults. Available from: Indian Health Services,

179

Headquarters West 300 San Mateo, NE, Suite 500
Albuquerque, NM 87108. Telephone: (505) 262–6112.

Morse, B.A. & Weiner, L. (1992)
FAS: Parent and Child
Fetal Alcohol Education Program, Brookline, MA

This booklet has been developed to help parents understand their child with fetal alcohol syndrome (FAS). Parents who recognize the reasons for their children's problems can plan the most effective treatment and educational strategies. This resource was designed with the help of the Massachusetts FAS Parents' Support Group. Contact: Fetal Alcohol Education Program, Boston University School of Medicine, 7 Kent Street, Brookline, MA 02146. Telephone: (617) 739–1424.

Secretary of Health and Human Services (1990)
*Fetal Alcohol Syndrome and Other Effects of Alcohol
  on Pregnancy Outcome*
Seventh Special Report to the U.S. Congress on Alcohol and Health (pp. 139–161) Rockville, MD

This chapter examines both fetal alcohol syndrome (FAS) and fetal alcohol effects (FAE). Research is reviewed on the effects of maternal alcohol consumption on pregnancy outcome with both clinical and animal research findings. Statistics are cited on the incidence of FAS and FAE in various demographic groups. An extensive bibliography is provided. Free of charge; write to: National Clearinghouse for Alcohol and Drug Information, P.O. Box 2345, Rockville, MD 20852. Maryland and D.C. Metro Area Call: (301) 468–2600 Toll free: 1(800) 729–6686.

U.S. Department of Health and Human Services (1990)
*Alcohol, Tobacco, and Other Drugs May Harm the
  Unborn*
Office for Substance Abuse Prevention
DIS Publication No. (ADM) 90–1711 Rockville, MD

Ultimately, this booklet is intended for women of child-bearing age and their partners. It is also written for health care providers and all others working with young women of childbearing age. It is addressed to volunteers active in the prevention and early intervention of drug abuse, including the abuse of beer, wine, distilled spirits, tobacco, and other drugs, be they illicit, prescribed, or over-the-counter. Available free from: National Clearinghouse for Alcohol and Drug Information, P.O. Box 2345, Rockville, MD 20852. In Maryland and D.C. Metro Area Call: (301) 468–2600. Toll free: 1 (800) 729–6686.

Johnson Institute Publications
(Various Titles)
Minneapolis, MN

The Johnson Institute is an internationally recognized leader in the field of chemical dependence intervention, treatment, and recovery for the past twenty years. A vast list of resources including publications, films, audio-cassettes, seminars, and special services, including training and consultation is available. Contact: Johnson Institute, 7151 Metro Blvd., Minneapolis, MN 55439. In Minneapolis/St. Paul call: 944-0511. Toll free in the U.S.: 1(800) 231–5165. In Canada: 1 (800) 447–6660. In Minnesota: 1 (800) 247–0484.

Newsletters

About the Various Newsletters: These newsletters all include articles written by parents and professionals who live and work with children with FAS/FAE, as well as updates on current research, books, and other educational materials. Progress made in legislation is announced, upcoming workshops on FAS/FAE are listed, and support groups are identified.

ICEBERG
P.O. Box 95597
Seattle, WA 98145-2597

A non-profit educational newsletter for people concerned about fetal alcohol syndrome and fetal alcohol effects, "because the problems we readily see are only the tip of the iceberg." Published quarterly; $10.00 family rate, $20.00 professional rate. Prepaid subscriptions only.

Growing with FAS
7802 SE Taylor
Portland, OR 97215

A fetal alcohol syndrome non-profit coalition publication; $4.00 for four issues.

FANN (Fetal Alcohol Network Newsletter)
158 Rosemont Avenue
Coatsville, PA 19320

This newsletter addresses issues of FAS/FAE, including lists of support groups, a telephone help line for contacting other parents, FAS/FAE meetings and conferences, etc. Write for subscription information.

Clearinghouse for Drug Exposed Children Newsletter
The Clearinghouse for Drug Exposed Children
Division of Behavioral and Developmental Pediatrics
University of California, San Francisco
400 Parnassus Avenue, Room A203
San Francisco,CA 94143–0314 (415) 476–9691

A national resource of available services for drug exposed children and families including community services, other publications, training programs, to name a few. A free publication.

ADAMHA News
(Alcohol, Drug Abuse, and Mental Health Administration)
U.S. Department of Health and Human Services
Public Health Service
Office of Communications and External Affairs

A concise, informative publication of research in the alcohol, drug abuse, and mental health fields. Includes the National Institute on Alcohol Abuse and Alcoholism (NIAAA), National Institute on Drug Abuse (NIDA), National Institute of Mental Health (NIMH), Office for Substance Abuse Prevention (OSAP), and Office for Treatment Improvement. Cost is $6.00 per year. Send prepaid subscriptions to: New Orders, Superintendent of Documents, P.O. Box 371954, Pittsburgh, PA 15250–7954.

F.A.S. Times
Fetal Alcohol Syndrome/Adolescent Task Force
Newsletter
P.O. Box 2525
Lynnwood, WA 98036

Family: $15 per year
Professional: $25 per year

FAS/E Newsletter
P.O. Box 74612
Fairbanks, AK 99707
(907) 456–1101

Teaching, Training, and Resource Materials

The Biomedical Aspects of Alcohol Use. Unit 5: Pregnancy and the Fetal Alcohol Syndrome.

Forty-six slides with 24 pages of text developed by the Project Cork Institute of Dartmouth Medical School, in cooperation with Milner-Fenwick. Authored by Ruth E. Little, Sc.D. and Ann P. Streissguth, Ph.D., $100.00.

A comprehensive and well-written unit illustrated with clear, concise charts, graphs and artwork. An excellent guide for community groups, learning resource centers, health department staff, alcohol treatment agencies and centers staff training, hospital staff, etc. Other alcohol-related slide units are available. Contact: Milner-Fenwick,

Inc., 2125 Greenspring, Dr. Timonium, MD 21093. Toll free: 1(800) 432–8433.

Alcohol and Other Drug Education and Prevention Materials

A catalog of materials from the University of Wisconsin-Madison appropriate for health professionals, schools, colleges, universities, teachers, students, parents, hospitals, community groups, etc. Includes posters, videos, books, pamphlets and other resources. Available from: Wisconsin Clearinghouse, P.O. Box 1468. Madison,WI 53701–1468. Toll free: 1 (800) 322–1468.

The F.A.S. Series

This series of four video tapes discusses the effects of alcohol on the fetus, the role that men play in encouraging women to drink, and primary and secondary prevention techniques for community, education, and health professionals. Strategies for assessing and dealing with the special needs of these children are discussed, as well as the problems they may face in the future. Titles: Program 1: "What is F.A.S.?"; Program 2: "Preventing F.A.S."; Program 3: "Assessment and the Early Years"; Program 4: "Adolescence and the Future." Previews are sent at no charge for purchase consideration. Contact: Perennial Education 930 Pitner Avenue, Evanston, IL 60202. Toll free: 1 (800) 323–9084.

Films and Videos for a Drug-Free Society

A catalog listing over 100 items on topics of education, prevention, intervention, early treatment, aftercare, DWDWL family education and HIV/AIDS awareness. These age-appropriate videos address tough issues in a sensitive, accurate and effective manner. Free previews; rent or purchase. Available from: AIMS Media, 9710 DeSoto Avenue, Chatsworth, CA 91311–4409. Toll free: 1 (800) 367–2467.

20/20 Transcript ($4.00)
FAS-March 1990
267 Broadway
New York, NY 10007
20/20 Video

Includes an excerpt on FAS that features Michael Dorris, author of *The Broken Cord,* Diane Malbin a therapist in private practice who counsels children with FAS and their families, Dr. Ann Streissguth, and Dr. Sterling Clarren. A number of children with FAS are interviewed, as are their parents, giving viewers an inside look at the way FAS affects these families' lives.

National Resource Centers

National Organization on Fetal Alcohol Syndrome
  (NOFAS)
1815 H Street, NW Suite 750
Washington, DC 20006
Telephone: 1–800–666–6327

Association for Retarded Citizens of the United States
  (ARC)
National ARC
500 East Border St., Third Floor
Arlington,TX 76010
Telephone: (817) 261–6003
Fax Number: (817) 277–3491
For further information contact your local ARC chapter.

National Clearinghouse for Alcohol and Drug
  Information (NCADI)
P.O. Box 2345
Rochester, MD 20852

National Institute on Alcohol Abuse and Alcoholism
  (NIAAA)
P.O. Box 2345
Rockville, MD 20852
Telephone: (301) 468–2600 / Toll free: 1 (800) 729–6686

NAPARE (National Association for Perinatal
   Addiction Research and Education)
11 E. Hubbard Street
Suite 200 Chicago, IL 60611
Telephone: (312) 329–9131
Toll free: NAPARE Alcohol, Drugs and Pregnancy
   Helpline: 1 (800) 638–2229

National Council on Alcoholism and Drug
   Dependence (NCADD)
12 West 21 Street
New York, NY 10010
Telephone: (212) 206–6770
Toll free Helpline: 1(800) 622–2255 or 1(800) 475–4673

National Perinatal Information Center
One State Street, Suite 102
Providence, RI 02908
Telephone: (401) 274–0650

Office for Substance Abuse Prevention (OSAP)
National Resource Center for the Prevention of
   Perinatal Abuse of Alcohol and Other Drugs
9300 Lee Highway
Fairfax, VA 22031
(703) 218–5600

March of Dimes Birth Defects Foundation
National Office Community Services Department
1275 Mamaroneck Avenue
White Plains, NY 10605
Telephone: (914) 428–7100
*For further information contact your local March of
   Dimes chapter.*

Children of Alcoholics Foundation
555 Madison Avenue
New York,NY 10022
Telephone: (212) 754–0656

National Association for Native American Children of
 Alcoholics
P.O. Box 18736
Seattle,WA 98118
Telephone: (206) 322–5601

National Association for Children of Alcoholics
31586 South Coast Hwy., Suite 201
South Laguna, CA 92677
Telephone: (714) 499–3899

National Black Alcoholism Council
1629 K Street, NW, Suite 802
Washington, DC 20006
Telephone: (202) 296–2696

Alcoholics Anonymous (AA)
National Chapter
P.O. Box 9999
Van Nuys, CA 91409
Telephone: (818) 780–3951

National Coalition for Hispanic Health & Human
 Services
1501 16th Street, NW
Washington, DC 20036
Telephone: (202) 387–5000
For further information contact your local AA chapter.

Adult Children of Alcoholics (ACOA)
P.O. Box 862
Midtown Station
New York, NY 10018
Toll free: 1(800) 344–2666

Al-Anon/Alateen Family Group Headquarters
P.O. Box 862, Midtown Station
New York, NY 10018
Telephone: (212) 351–9500

If you want to talk to someone about a problem with alcohol or drugs, call toll free: 1 (800) 662–4357.

Adopted Child
P.O. Box 9362
Moscow, ID 83843

National Information Center for Children and Youth
  with Handicaps
P.O. Box 1492
Washington, DC 20013

National Institute of Alcohol Abuse and Alcoholism
5600 Fishers Lane
Rockville, MD 20857

Cocaine Baby Help Line
1–800–327–BABE

Fetal Alcohol Education Program
Boston University School of Medicine
7 Kent Street
Brookline, MA 02146

Parent Support Groups

Parents Helping Parents
535 Race Street
Suite 220
San Jose, CA 95126
(408) 288–5010

Adolescent Autonomy Project
Children's Rehab Center
2270 Ivy Road
Charlottesville, VA 22901
(804) 294–8184

Pamela Groves
7802 Taylor
Portland, OR 97215
(503) 292–4056

Marceil Ten Eyck
1029 Market Street
Suite C2
Kirkland, WA 98033

Additional Resources

Black, Claudia. *It Will Never Happen to Me,* New York, Ballantine Books, 1981.

Bradshaw, John. *The Family,* Florida, Health Communications, Inc.

Dorris, Michael. *The Broken Cord,* New York, Harper & Row, 1989.

Glinta, Carole T., Ann P. Streissguth. "Patients with Fetal Alcohol Syndrome and Their Caretakers," *Social Casework: The Journal of Contemporary Social Work,* 1988, pp. 453–459.

Groves, Pamela G. "Effectively Dealing with Fetal Alcohol Syndrome, *The Counselor,* November/December, 1990, pp. 18-19.

Jones, K.l. and D.W. Smith. "Recognition of the Fetal Alcohol Syndrome in Early Infancy," *Lancet,* 1:1973, pp. 999–1001.

Milam, James R., K. Ketcham. *Under The Influence,* New York, Bantam Books, 1981.

Royce, James. *Alcohol Problems and Alcoholism,* New York, The Free Press, 1981.

Satir, Virginia. *Making Contact,* California, Celestial Arts, 1976.

Streissguth, Ann P., Robin A LaDue. "Fetal Alcohol: Teratogenic Causes of Developmental Disabilities," *Toxic*

Substances and Mental Retardation, Washington D.C., American Association on Mental Deficiency, pp. 1–32, 1987.

Villarreal, Sylvia F., Lora-Ellen McKinney, Marcia Quackenbush. *Handle with Care,* California, ETR Assoc., 1992.

Weinberg, Joanne. "Prenatal Ethanol Exposure Alters Adrenocortical Development of Offspring," *Alcoholism: Clinical and Experimental Research,* February 1989, Vol. 13, pp. 73–82.

NOTES

NOTES

NOTES

NOTES

NOTES

NOTES

NOTES

NOTES

NOTES

NOTES

NOTES